the *NEW!*
Abs
Diet
for Women

the NEW! Abs Diet for Women

The 6-Week Plan to Flatten Your Belly and Firm Up Your Body for Life

DAVID ZINCZENKO

EDITORIAL DIRECTOR of Women'sHealth

With Ted Spiker

RODALE

Some portions of this book have appeared previously in *Men's Health*, *Prevention*, and *Women's Health* magazines.

Published as direct mail hardcover in 2010, trade hardcover in 2011, and trade paperback in 2012.

Rodale books may be purchased for business or promotional use or for special sales. For information, please write to:

Special Markets Department, Rodale Inc., 733 Third Avenue, New York, NY 10017

The Abs Diet, Men's Health, and *Women's Health* are registered trademarks of Rodale Inc.

Printed in the United States of America
Rodale Inc. makes every effort to use acid-free ♾, recycled paper ♻.

Photographs by Mitch Mandel and Beth Bischoff

Illustrations by L-Dopa

Book design by Joe Heroun and Courtney Eltringham, with George Karabotsos, design director, *Men's Health* Books and *Women's Health* Books

Library of Congress Cataloging-in-Publication Data

Zinczenko, David.
  The abs diet for women : the six-week plan to flatten your belly and firm up your body for life / David Zinczenko with Ted Spiker.
     p.   cm.
  Includes index.
  ISBN-13: 978-1-60529-275-5 (direct hardcover)
  ISBN-13: 978-1-60529-315-8 (trade hardcover)
  ISBN-13: 978-1-60961-384-6 (trade paperback)
1. Reducing exercises.   2. Abdominal exercises.   3. Reducing diets.
4. Exercise for women.   I. Spiker, Ted.   II. Title.
RA781.6.Z58   2007
613.7'12—dc22
                                     2007004035

2 4 6 8 10 9 7 5 3 1   trade paperback

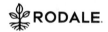

RODALE.

We inspire and enable people to improve their lives and the world around them.

www.theAbsDiet.com

*For women everywhere who know
how much we love, need, and admire them:
Here's the next step to a
happier, healthier, fitter you.*

CONTENTS

FOREWORD

GET THE BODY YOU WANT, WITHOUT SACRIFICING THE THINGS YOU LOVE

I HAVE A FRIEND WHO DREADS going to parties because she equates socializing with overeating. Imagine that—she would rather skip spending time with her friends than put herself in harm's way of circulating appetizer trays carrying tempting bites.

She's not alone, of course. I can relate. I'm sure you can, too. Is there something in the female DNA that compels us to beat ourselves up the day after enjoying a slice of cheesecake or a few mini hamburger sliders?

Perhaps we mistake the power of food for a character flaw. Unless we are denying ourselves one of life's basic pleasures—eating delicious food—we can't feel good about who we are or how we look in our jeans. Yet denial is not a sustainable eating strategy. It's against human nature to deprive ourselves and, frankly, it's not a fun way to get ready for bikini season!

That's why I'm so excited about this new edition of the bestselling *Abs Diet for Women.* Four years ago, David Zinczenko, senior vice president and editor-in-chief of *Men's Health,* penned this revolutionary eating guide to address the unique challenges women face when it comes to losing weight. And it has helped hundreds of thousands of women just like you and me to improve their health. What makes this diet so refreshing is that it's not about sacrifice. It's not about what you can't eat. It doesn't require monitoring every morsel that passes your lips. Instead, the Abs Diet for Women puts you in control of your fitness and nutrition: eat the right food (and more of it!) and you'll trim away belly fat for good. And though this diet was designed specifically to give you a flat tummy, your whole body will benefit from the fat-torching eating and exercise plans.

The secret weight-loss method detailed in *The New Abs Diet for Women* involves the Power 12, a cornucopia of foods that will fill you up, satisfy your hunger longer, and help power up your body's natural fat burners. Make these foods the focus of your meals and snacks—at home, at work, at parties and when you travel—and you won't ever have to count calories. You'll never again feel guilty about eating great food.

This, *The New Abs Diet for Women,* has been updated with the latest nutrition research, fantastic new recipes using the 12 Abs Diet Powerfoods, and fast-acting, fat-blasting exercises. And we couldn't be launching it at a more critical time. Our nation is facing a major health crisis. More than 142 million Americans are obese or overweight. More than 10 percent of all women age 20 or older are living with diabetes, a devastating, life-threatening disease. Telling people to just say no to fast food or fat or carbs has not worked. Providing people with the tools to take charge of their health will. And that's what the New Abs Diet for Women does, brilliantly.

So grab a jar of natural peanut butter (it's an Abs Diet Powerfood!). Lace up your walking (or running!) shoes and try the new metabolism-boosting workout on page 219. Soon you'll be on your way to a healthier, hotter body for life. You deserve it!

—Michele Promaulayko, editor-in-chief of *Women's Health*

INTRODUCTION

YOUR ABS MAY SAVE YOUR LIFE
You Have Abs. Yes, You.
And This Plan Will Help You Find Them

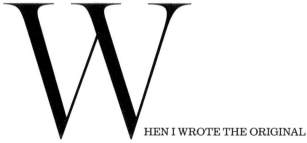

WHEN I WROTE THE ORIGINAL *Abs Diet* more than 5 years ago, some people thought it was written for beach volleyball players, body-builders, and people who aspire to prance around in front of large-format cameras wearing lace thongs. It couldn't possibly be for real men and women who have more pressing things to do than crunch washboard bellies in a gym all day long.

But then a funny thing happened. It wasn't the athletes or rappers or Victoria's Secret models who picked up the book, but tens of thousands of real men and women. People like you. They gave the program a shot, lost the stubborn pounds, found their hidden abdominal muscles, and, most important, dramatically improved their health.

Then they told their friends about it. And that's how *The Abs Diet* became a *New York Times* bestseller and spawned a half dozen other books, including *The New Abs Diet Cookbook* released in 2010.

I'm proud of the Abs Diet and the impact it has made on people's lives. But I'm not satisfied. Not yet, because so many more people still need to hear the message and learn the secrets to losing weight and firming up their bodies for life. I know that some critics see flat bellies as the modern American symbol of vanity, but dropping pounds, inches and dress sizes is more than just a way to support the mirror industry. We are at a crucial point in our nation's history: We're too darned fat. Obesity has overtaken smoking as the leading cause of premature heart attacks in the United States. Imagine that—overeating is worse for you than smoking a pack a day. We've forced the smokers out of our restaurants and onto the sidewalk to light up, and yet you can still order an appetizer off the menu that delivers a day's worth of calories and enough grease to turn your colon into a Roman candle. Go figure.

Sixty-seven percent of the population—roughly 142 million Americans—are overweight or obese. And a new forecast by University of Chicago researchers estimates that the number of Americans living with diabetes will nearly double in the next 25 years to 44.1 million people.

But it doesn't have to be that way. And I know that the Abs Diet can help. So, whether you are worried about pre-diabetes or your cholesterol numbers, or you're just a little anxious about the approaching bikini season, here's my promise: With this book you will improve your health and find your abs, and if I can also help you into that barely-there bathing suit, well then I'm happy to oblige.

As the editor-in-chief of *Men's Health* magazine, and editorial director of *Women's Health,* I know that you—no matter how flabby your belly, how many kids you've brought into this world, or how many diets you've tried—can develop a flat stomach. See, I analyze health and fitness information with the time and tenacity that your boyfriends and husbands devote to their fantasy baseball teams. It's my job to find the fastest, best and smartest ways for you to make tremendous gains in your most important investment: your body. And I'm encouraged by all the new research in nutrition and exercise science in the past 5 years, amazing strategies you'll put into practice later in the book. A flat stomach—that is, abs that show—is a worthy goal because it's the ultimate predictor of your health. And you will get there even if you've failed on previous weight-loss attempts and have yo-yoed more than kids at a toy store. I understand your struggle. I've talked to and heard from thousands of women who have shared their weight-loss attempts with me. I know what you've gone through because I, too, know what it's like to feel fat.

As a latchkey kid growing up in the early '80s, I made every mistake in the book. I ate fast food instead of smart food. I played video games when I should've been playing outside. By the time I reached 14, I was carrying 212 pounds of torpid teenage tallow on my 5-foot-10 frame. I wanted to be built like a basketball player, but instead I was built like the basketball. And I paid for it with a steady bombardment of humiliation. My older brother, Eric, would invite friends to our house just to watch me eat lunch. "Don't disturb the big animal," he'd tell his friends. "It's feeding."

Like most kids, I learned my health habits from my parents, particularly my father. He was more than 100 pounds overweight for most of his adult life. Over time, he developed hypertension and diabetes, had a minor heart attack, and would have to stop at the top of a short flight of stairs just to catch his breath. A massive stroke ended his life at 52. My father died because he ignored many signals of failing health—especially the fat that padded his gut.

But I got lucky. When I graduated from high school, I joined the Naval Reserve, where the tenets of fitness were pounded into me, day after day after day. Soon after I graduated from college, I joined *Men's Health* and learned the importance of proper nutrition and—just as important—the danger of carrying around too much fat in your stomach.

Belly fat—the fat that pushes your waist out—is the most dangerous fat on your body. And it's one of the reasons why the Abs Diet emphasizes losing belly fat: because doing so means you'll live longer. Belly fat is classified as visceral fat; that means it is located behind your abdominal wall and surrounds your internal organs. Because it carries an express-lane pass to your heart and other important organs, visceral fat is the fat that can kill you. Just consider one University of Alabama–Birmingham study in which researchers used seven different measurements to determine a person's risks of cardiovascular disease. They concluded that the amount of visceral fat the subjects carried was the single best predictor of heart disease risk.

Whether you want to change your body to improve your health, your looks, your energy levels, or your sex appeal, the Abs Diet for Women offers you a simple promise: If you follow this plan, you will transform your body so that you can accomplish each and every one of those goals. As a bonus, the Abs Diet will do something more than just enhance your life; the Abs Diet is going to save it.

And in this special edition, *The New Abs Diet for Women*, you'll do more than transform your body into a lean one. You'll also learn how to make the Abs Diet principles work for you specifically—considering your lifestyle, your hormones, and the fact that many of you have to deal with the one biological factor that men don't have to consider: Your belly is stretched not only by sour cream and key lime pie but also by little runts that like to nestle in there for 9 months at a time.

|||||||||||||||||||||||||||||||||||||||||||||||||||||||||||||||||||||||||||||||||||||||||||||||||||||||||||||||||

Diet Is a Four-Letter Word

In all honesty, I hated to even call this book a "diet" book. That's because the word *diet* has been twisted around to mean something you follow temporarily—you "go on a diet." But if you "go on" a diet, you eventually have to "go off" it. And that's why most diets are really, really bad for you.

Most diets are about eating less food or about restricting you to certain kinds of food. Most of them work in the short term because if you reduce your calorie intake, your body starts to burn itself off in order to keep itself alive. Presto, you lose weight. But here's the problem: The first thing your body does when it's short of calories is to dump the body tissue that takes the most calories to maintain.

That's muscle. So on a low-calorie diet, your body burns away muscle and tries to store fat. Sure, you'll lose weight, and you'll eventually start losing fat as well. But when you "go off" your diet, you'll start to put weight back on. And guess what kind of weight you'll gain? Pure fat. Because you've taught your body a harsh lesson: It has to be on the lookout for potential low-calorie periods in the future, so it had better store fat just in case. You've also used up valuable calorie-burning muscle, so you're likely to end up fatter than you were before your diet. That's why people who try diet after diet not only don't lose weight but also gain it.

The Abs Diet isn't a shotgun, irresponsible approach to weight management. Oh, you'll lose weight, and you'll lose it fast. But you'll lose fat, not muscle. And you'll keep that weight off for life. You'll follow the tenets of the Abs Diet for life, too, because it's about eating lots and lots of great food in smart ways. So enjoy the Abs Diet. But let's keep that little four-letter word between us, okay?

When you think of all you have to gain with the Abs Diet, it becomes apparent what's wrong with most diet plans out there: They're all about losing. When you consider America's obesity epidemic, losing weight is an admirable goal. But I think there's a fundamental psychological reason why many of these diets fail: There's no motivation in losing. Americans don't like to lose. We don't like to lose board games. We don't like to lose in the market. We don't like to lose our smooth skin, our teeth, or our bodies' fight against gravity. We don't like to lose anything. In a way, we don't even like losing weight because we've all been force-fed the notion that bigger is better. Instead, we're programmed to gain. We want to gain fitness. We want to gain strength. We want to add to our life, not subtract from it. We want to win—and see our results. So consider the Abs Diet a shift in the way you think about your body and about weight loss. This program concentrates on what you can gain and how you can gain it. As a result of what you'll gain from this program—abs, muscle tone, energy, better health, a great sex life (more on that later)—you'll effortlessly strip away fat from your body and change your body shape forever.

No diet plan would work without good nutrition, so that, of course, is the major focus of the Abs Diet. You'll not only learn what to eat, you'll also learn how to eat to make your body burn fat furiously, as well as how to make sure that you can control the cravings that threaten to add girth to your middle. The focus of the plan revolves around—but does not restrict you to—12 "Powerfoods" that are among the best sources of protein, fiber, and all the other ingredients and nutrients that help fight fat. When you build your diet around these foods, you will build a new body in the process. But we've taken this weight-loss plan to a whole other level. While nutrition remains a principal component of most diets, too many programs out there focus solely on how to change your eating habits—cut carbs, add cabbage soup, eat at Subway twice a day. Those programs fail to recognize a crucial component of weight control: the fact that our bodies have their own natural fat-burning mechanism . . .

Muscle.

BUILDING JUST A FEW POUNDS of muscle in your body is the physiological equivalent of kicking fat out on its butt and telling it to never come back again. Muscle—in the form of lean muscle mass, not bulky, bodybuilder muscle mass—exponentially speeds up the fat-busting process: One pound of muscle requires your body to burn up to 50 extra calories a day just to maintain that muscle. Now think about what happens if you add just a few pounds of toned muscle over the course of a diet program. It'll take your body up to several hundred extra calories a day just to feed that muscle—essentially, you'll burn off an extra pound of fat every few weeks without doing a thing (and that's not even including the gains you can make by changing your diet). When you combine exercise with the foods that most promote lean muscle growth, the ones that keep you full, and the ones that give your body a well-balanced supply of nutrients, you'll be in the sweet spot, doing what this plan is all about.

You'll change the shape of your body by stripping your fat and showing off your lean muscle.

Does that mean the Abs Diet is going to make you burly, muscle-bound, or governor of California? Not at all. The Abs Diet for Women and the accompanying Abs Diet Workout emphasize leanness and muscle tone—not big, mannish muscles.

Going back to that important investment, you can think about muscle as your compound interest. If you've ever taken a basic economics course, then you understand how compound interest works: If you invest $100 in a high-yield fund and add a little more every month, over time that investment will grow and grow to half a million dollars or more. But you'll have invested only a fraction of the money yourself. Compound interest is what allows you to make the most dramatic financial gains. It's the same concept with your body. Invest in a little additional muscle in the next 6 weeks—through eating the right foods and following a muscle-adding, fat-burning exercise plan—and you'll have invested in a lean and strong body that can last a lifetime because your new muscle will continually break down fat to stay alive.

I'm passionate about this plan because I know it works. I've seen it work, and so will you. During the course of this 6-week plan, you can lose up to 20 pounds of fat (much of it in the first couple of weeks, and from your belly first) and gain several pounds of lean muscle. But the biggest thing you'll notice is that you'll have significantly changed the shape of your body. Some of you will have even more dramatic results (see page 30 for the story of Linda Toomey, who lost 16 pounds in the first 6 weeks on the diet and cut her body fat percentage from 36 to 25). The Abs Diet includes all three components to a successful body-transforming program: nutrition, exercise, and the motivational principles to follow through. I've designed this program to make it easy to stick to, even if you've tried and failed with diets in the past. It's easy to follow because:

▶ Every component of the diet and exercise plan is quick, simple, and flexible enough so that you can easily work it into your life.

▶ Every goal is attainable.

▶ Every principle is supported by well-respected scientific research.

The Abs Diet will change the way you think about your body. It's the first plan to count not just the calories your body takes in but the calories your body burns off as well. Using the most cutting-edge nutrition and exercise research, the Abs Diet will show you how to retrain your body to burn fat faster and more efficiently—even while you sleep—and to focus your meals around the foods that inspire your body to keep those calorie-burning fires stoked. The Abs Diet isn't about counting calories (though you certainly can if that works for you); it's about making your calories count.

Throughout the book, I'll take you through the principles of the Abs Diet and show you how to follow the 6-week plan. I'll also explain the exercise program (which doesn't have to start until the 3rd week) and give you instructions on how to perform the exercises and how to make the meals. (For the time-crunched, you can cook up many of our Powerfood feasts with only a blender.)

To keep you motivated, I've included the stories of real-life women who credit the Abs Diet with changing their bodies and their lives—not to mention their wardrobes.

THE ABS DIET CHEAT SHEET

(And Portion-Distortion Decoder)

HERE'S AN AT-A-GLANCE guide that summarizes the principles of the Abs Diet: the 6-week plan to flatten your belly and firm up your body for life. New for this edition, I've added a handy serving-size decoder because I've learned through talking with many female and male veterans of this program that portion control is another useful tool for Abs Diet success.

ABS DIET CHEAT SHEET

HABIT	GUIDELINE
EAT	6 meals (including snacks) spaced evenly throughout the day.
PLAN	most meals around the **ABS DIET POWER 12** food groups. Each meal should contain at least two of the following:

A lmonds and other nuts
B eans and legumes
S pinach and other green vegetables

D airy (fat-free or low-fat milk, yogurt, cheese)
I nstant oatmeal (unsweetened, unflavored)
E ggs
T urkey and other lean meats

P eanut butter
O live oil
W hole-grain breads and cereals
E xtra-protein (whey) powder
R aspberries and other berries

EMPHASIZE	protein, fiber, calcium, and healthy fats (mono- and polyunstaturated).
LIMIT	refined carbohydrates such as baked goods, sugar, white bread, rice and pasta, saturated fats, trans fats, and high-fructose corn syrup.

HABIT	GUIDELINE
DRINK	mostly water. Limit yourself to two or three alcoholic beverages per week to maximize the benefits of the Abs Diet plan.
CHEAT	once a week by eating anything your heart desires.
EXERCISE	for 20 minutes 3 days a week during weeks 3 through 6 of the program. Exercise is optional for the first 2 weeks, but brisk walking is highly recommended. Total-body strength workouts that can be done at the gym or at home, as well as new interval training programs, are detailed in this book. Two of your strength-training workouts should contain exercises that work your abdominals.

ABS DIET PORTION-DISTORTION DECODER

PORTION	ABOUT EQUAL TO...
3 ounces lean meat or poultry	deck of playing cards
3 ounces fish	checkbook
2 tablespoons peanut butter	golf ball
1 tablespoon salad dressing	poker chip
1 ounce hard cheese	3 stacked dice
1 ounce mozzarella cheese	Ping-Pong ball
1 tablespoon butter or mayonnaise	poker chip
1 cup chili or yogurt	baseball
1 serving popcorn	3 baseballs
1 baked potato	computer mouse
1 medium fruit	baseball
1 serving almonds	¼ cup or 12 almonds
1 serving pistachios	¼ cup or 24 pistachios
1 serving sausage	shotgun shell
1 serving (½ cup) ice cream	tennis ball
4 ounces dried spaghetti	diameter of a quarter when held tightly and viewed from end
½ cup cooked spaghetti	tight fist
8 ounce serving of lasagna	2 hockey pucks

Chapter 1

THE NEXT STEP IN WEIGHT LOSS
Cutting-Edge Research Blazes New Paths to a Flat Belly and Healthy Body

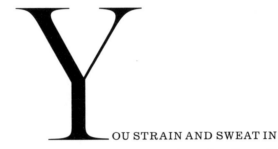 OU STRAIN AND SWEAT IN
cardio class, but that belly flab won't budge. Maybe you stepped on the scale
today and were shocked to find that you're heavier than you were two days ago
despite a week of eating every conceivable variation of soy and celery.

What gives? My guess is you've been going about weight loss the wrong way.
But don't beat yourself up; it's not your fault. You've been conditioned to fight
your body's natural fat burners through diets of denial that leave you coveting
your co-worker's meatball sandwich. You've been disappointed by the work-
out-of-the-stars du jour, which leaves you feeling sore and frustrated. You've
been misled into thinking that there's some magic bullet out there that's going
to finally give you the body you want, if only you could put up with the sacrifice
and torture for a few weeks.

I have an option for you that's not so painful: take your cues from people
who make it their life's work to study weight loss, nutrition, and fitness. The
Abs Diet for Women is based on the latest studies from research hospitals and
university labs. In the 5 years since we first published the Abs Diet books,

much new research has been done that further supports its core principles and suggests ways to make it even more effective.

Let's review some of the breakthroughs in nutrition and exercise science that, as you will see, dovetail very nicely with the core tenets of the Abs Diet for Women fitness and weight loss program. I guarantee they will open your eyes and motivate you to start living the Abs Diet lifestyle today.

|||||||||||||||||||||||||||||||||||||||||||||||||||||||||||||||||||||||||||||||||||||||||||||||||||||||||||||||||

Big Numbers

Overweight people are:

▶ 50 percent more likely to develop heart disease
(obese: up to 100 percent)

▶ Up to 360 percent more likely to develop diabetes
(obese: up to 1,020 percent)

▶ 16 percent more likely to die of a first heart attack (obese: 49 percent)

▶ Roughly 50 percent more likely to have total cholesterol above
250 (obese: up to 122 percent)

▶ 14 percent less attractive to the opposite sex (obese: 43 percent)

▶ Likely to spend 37 percent more a year at the pharmacy
(obese: 105 percent)

▶ Likely to stay 19 percent longer in the hospital (obese: 49 percent)

▶ 20 percent more likely to have asthma (obese: 50 percent)

▶ Up to 31 percent more likely to die of any cause (obese: 62 percent)

▶ 19 percent more likely to die in a car crash (obese: 37 percent)

▶ 120 percent more likely to develop stomach cancer (obese: 330 percent)

▶ Up to 90 percent more likely to develop gallstones
(obese: up to 150 percent)

▶ 590 percent more likely to develop esophageal cancer
(obese: 1,520 percent)

▶ 35 percent more likely to develop kidney cancer (obese: 70 percent)

▶ 14 percent more likely to have osteoarthritis (obese: 34 percent)

▶ 70 percent more likely to develop high blood pressure
(obese: up to 170 percent)

What you eat NOW has a profound affect on what you'll eat LATER.

▶ Scientists at the USDA Human Nutrition Research Center at Tufts University found that eating foods that elevate your blood sugar trigger intense cravings for carbohydrates later on. In other words, eating a cookie begets eating more cookies and so on. Eating carbohydrates such as baked goods and pasta or sugary foods, they say, promotes greater calorie consumption, not just now, but during the rest of the day.

▶ In 2008, the *British Journal of Nutrition* reported that consuming high-quality protein early in the day results in more sustained fullness compared with eating similar meals in the evening.

▶ A similar study at Purdue University found that men on a calorie-restricted diet had their hunger satisfied the longest when they were given extra protein at breakfast.

Certain foods may boost metabolism and target belly fat.

As you'll see, the Abs Diet program encourages you to try to eat protein with every meal and snack. Protein is recommended for several reasons. It fills you up, it digests more slowly than fast-absorbing carbs do, it spurs lean muscle growth, and it even elevates fat burn, as research continues to prove.

▶ A study in the *International Journal of Obesity* determined that eating two eggs in the morning promotes weight loss. In the experiment, overweight subjects ate a 340-calorie breakfast of either two eggs or a single bagel 5 days a week for 8 weeks. Those who ate these inexpensive protein-packed wonders, the study found, lost 65 percent more weight than the bagel eaters, with no effect on their cholesterol or triglyceride levels.

▶ Whole grains work, too. A 2009 study in the *American Journal of Clinical Nutrition* showed that a calorie-controlled diet rich in whole grains trimmed extra fat from the waistline of obese subjects. Study participants who ate all whole grains (in addition to five servings of fruits and vegetables, three servings of low-fat dairy, and two servings of lean meat, fish, or poultry) lost more weight from the abdominal area than another group that ate the same diet, but with all refined grains.

▶ Another new study in the journal *Obesity* finds that people who eat nuts just twice a week are about 30 percent less likely to gain weight than people who rarely eat nuts. Similar research from the City of Home National Medical Center in Duarte, California, determined that dieters who ate a few ounces of almonds every day lost

||||||||||||||||||||||||||||||||||||||||||||||||||||||||||||||||||||||||||||||||||||||||||||||||||||||||||||

Six-Pack Secrets

Weigh yourself. Checking the scale can be motivating. In a study of 3,500 people who maintained 60 or more pounds of weight loss for at least a year, researchers from the National Weight Control Registry found that 44 percent weighed themselves every day. Another study in the *American Journal of Preventive Medicine* found that overweight people are six times more likely to lose weight if they weigh themselves at least once a day.

Eat, then write. People who kept a food diary lost twice as much weight as those who didn't, according to a study of 1,685 overweight or obese adults at Kaiser Permanente Center for Health Research.

Walk to the water fountain. An Australian study showed that workers who sat for more than 6 hours a day were up to 68 percent more likely to be overweight or obese than those who sat less. The take-home advice: Get out of your chair and move around more. If you work on a computer all day, consider raising the screen and keyboard so that you can stand and do your work.

Leave something on your plate. Cleaning your plate makes for large bellies. In a Cornell University survey, researchers found that the heaviest participants said they stopped eating not when they felt full but when they made a significant dent in what they thought was a normal-sized plate of food.

Chew, chew, chew chew. Dutch researchers found that people who chewed large bites of food for 3 seconds consumed 52 percent more food before feeling full than those who chewed smaller bites for 9 seconds. Eating slower and talking between swallows also reduces calorie consumption, studies show.

6½ inches from their waists in 24 weeks, 50 percent more than dieters who ate the same number of calories without the fiber-rich nuts.

Diet and exercise work better than exercise alone.

▶ A combination order of whole grains and regular exercise adds up to greater belly-fat loss. In a study conducted by researchers at Pennsylvania State University, 50 obese subjects were split into two groups. One group was instructed to eat whole grains as their only grain choices; the other was told to avoid whole grains. Both groups were encouraged to do moderate exercise. After 12 weeks, the exercisers who ate whole grains lost a significantly larger percentage of belly fat than those who ate refined grains. Furthermore, their levels of C-reactive protein, a warning signal of heart disease and diabetes, had dropped by 38 percent, while the people who avoided whole-grain foods saw no change in their CRP levels.

▶ A 2008 study at the Human Performance Laboratory at the University of Connecticut suggests a similar strategy for triggering the body to burn more fat. In an experiment, two groups of men were instructed to do resistance training while following either a low-carbohydrate or low-fat diet. After 12 weeks, the lifters who reduced their intake of carbohydrates lost an average of 17 pounds of fat, twice as much as the lifters who followed the low-fat plan. What's more, each member of the low-carb group gained about 2 pounds of lean muscle. "Restricting carbohydrates forces your body to burn fat instead of sugar," says study author and assistant professor Jeff Volek, Ph.D. And doing so will work as effectively for you as it did for the men in this particular study. The eating plan in this book will show you exactly how to reduce consumption of empty carbs and properly fuel your body for a metabolic lift.

▶ Eating a breakfast of slow-burning carbohydrates such as oats can significantly improve calorie-burn during exercise, according to a study at the University of Nottingham reported in 2009 in the *Journal of Nutrition*. When active women were given a breakfast of low-glycemic index foods 3 hours before embarking on a 60-minute run, the amount of fat they burned during exercise was 55 percent higher than when they ate a high-carb, high-glycemic breakfast. Are you seeing my point?

Protein is a dieter's friend

▶ Recently, British researchers measured the effect of eating a protein-rich snack after a workout versus a high-carbohydrate snack: Those who consumed 43 grams of protein in a low-carb snack burned 21 percent more fat than the subjects who chugged a sugary post-workout drink. Not only do you expend more energy processing protein than carbs, but the amino acids in protein may lower levels of the stress hormone cortisol in your blood, which could boost your metabolic rate, say scientists at Syracuse University.

Food is powerful medicine

▶ Italian researchers found that eating as little as 1 cup of raw vegetables daily can add 2 years to your life. What does raw have to do with it? They say that cooking depletes up to 30 percent of the disease-fighting antioxidants in vegetables. Here's a quick way to get your quota: Fill a ziplock bag with chopped red and green peppers, broccoli, and carrots, and toss them into your work bag with a packet of dressing for an easy lunch. The fat in the dressing will boost your body's absorption of certain nutrients.

▶ Green tea may help exercisers burn more belly fat, according to a new 2009 study from the American Society of Nutrition. The 12-week study showed that subjects who drank green tea and did 180 minutes of moderately intense exercise per week lost twice as much weight as people who exercised but didn't drink the catechinrich beverage. The green-tea group also had larger declines in total abdominal fat, subcutaneous abdominal fat and triglycerides.

▶ When researchers at Loma Linda University tracked the eating habits of 34,000 Seventh-Day Adventists—a population famous for its longevity—they discovered that those who ate nuts (an Abs Diet Powerfood!) 5 days a week tended to outlive those who didn't eat nuts by 3 years. Scientists believe the monounsaturated fats and fiber in the nuts provide a longevity benefit and help keep weight in check.

▶ A new report by Duke University researchers shows that patients who have nonalcoholic fatty liver disease, a problem in which excess blood sugar converts to fat in your liver, can actually reverse their disease by making easy dietary changes. Simply by swapping in whole grains and fruits for fast-absorbing sugars and starches, the people in the study were able to lose weight and eliminate visceral fat deposits from around their liver.

Exercise is the best medicine

▶ When researchers tracked the walking habits of 1,300 women for 8 years, they discovered that the faster walkers had a lower death rate than the slower walkers and used fewer medications for diabetes, high blood pressure and high cholesterol, according to the *Journal of Nutrition, Health, and Aging*.

▶ A 2009 Arizona State University review of studies examining the effects of exercise on depression found that people who participated in exercise treatment had significantly lower depression scores than clinically depressed people who did not exercise.

▶ Strength training for 4 days a week for 13 weeks decreased lower back pain in chronic sufferers by nearly 30 percent, according to a recent report given at the American College of Sports Medicine annual meeting.

▶ Two other fitness related studies show that regular exercise relieves constipation in people with irritable bowel syndrome and cigarette cravings in ex-smokers.

▶ Do you think that physicians might do us a favor by prescribing more exercise and fewer drugs? I do.

How you work out is more important than how long you exercise

NEW RESEARCH DONE in the years since we first published *The Abs Diet for Women* supports the idea that high-intensity workouts are the most effective for reducing belly fat.

▶ One recent study at the University of Arkansas demonstrated that exercisers who did shorter, high-intensity workouts had a 20 percent reduction in dangerous visceral (deep abdominal) fat after 3 months compared with no change in people who did longer workouts at moderate pace. Researchers say that alternating short bursts of fast walking with slower segments can burn an average of 25 percent more calories.

▶ A Penn State University study found that people who lifted weights while following a program of diet and aerobic exercise had the same weight loss as those who only dieted (or who dieted and performed aerobic exercise). The difference? The lifters lost 5 pounds more fat because almost none of their weight loss came from losing muscle.

▶ A 2009 study at the University of Oklahoma found that people following a resistance-training workout three times a week for 14 weeks experienced significant improvements in weight loss, waist circumference and the greatest decreases in fasting insulin levels.

▶ Another new study demonstrated the belly-fat-frying benefit of adding weight training to a vigorous walking or jogging routine. In the 12-week experiment at Skidmore College, exercisers who did a high-intensity total-body resistance workout along with cardio lost four times as much belly fat when compared with exercisers who only did cardio workouts. The researchers attribute the extra fat loss to two things: the stepped-up calorie burn you get immediately after lifting weights and later when you increase your lean muscle mass. Whenever you lose weight, it typically comes from both fat and muscle tissue. Resistance training helps you maintain muscle, which prevents a slowdown in your metabolism.

Why it's important to lose that belly

NOW THAT YOU'VE had a glimpse of the new research that's going to help you find your abs, let's learn why abs are so important to a healthy body. We'll begin with a quick biology review:

The average American is carrying around about 30 billion fat cells. Each of those buggers is is filled with greasy substances called lipids. When you pump doughnuts, corn chips, and fried Snickers bars into your system, those fat cells can expand—up to 1,000 times their original size. But a fat cell can get only so big; once it reaches its physical limit, it starts to behave like a long-running sitcom. It creates spin-offs, leaving you with two or more fat cells for the price of one. Only problem: Fat cells have a no-return policy. Once you have a fat cell, you're stuck with it. So as you grow fatter and double the number of fat cells in your body, you also double the difficulty you'll have losing the lipids inside them.

Many of us tend to store fat in our bellies, and that's where the health dangers of excess weight begin. Some of us store it above the belt, while others store it below the belt. In any case, abdominal fat doesn't just sit there and do nothing; it's active. It functions like a separate organ, releasing substances that can be harmful to your body. For instance, it releases free fatty acids that impair your ability to break down the hormone insulin (too much insulin in your system can lead to diabetes). Fat also secretes substances that increase your risk of heart attacks and strokes, as well as the stress hormone cortisol (high levels of cortisol are also associated with diabetes, obesity, and high blood pressure). Abdominal fat bears the blame for many health problems because it resides within striking distance of your heart, liver, and other organs—pressing on them, feeding them poisons, and messing with their daily function.

Now take a look at the people with flat stomachs and six-packs. They're the icons of strength and good health. They're lean; they're strong; they look good in clothes; they look good without clothes. A defined midsection, in many ways, has defined fitness. But it also defines something else: A flat stomach is the hallmark of people in control of their bodies and, as such, in control of their health.

While some people may think that working toward a flat belly is shallower than a kiddie pool, there's nothing wrong with striving for a flat stomach or a defined midsection. Of course, defined abs make you look good—and make others feel good about the way you look, too. (In one survey, both men and women rated abs as the sexiest body part.) And for good reason: When you're in great shape, you're telling the world that you're a disciplined, motivated, confident, and healthy person—and hence a desirable partner. And as you've seen above, sometimes a little vanity can be good for your health. Here's more evidence: A Canadian study of more than 8,000 people found that over 13 years, the people with the weakest abdominal muscles had a death rate more than twice as high of those with the strongest midsections. Such research upholds the notion that flat stomachs do more than turn heads at the beach. In fact, your abdominal muscles control more of your body than you may even realize—and have just as much substance as show. In short, here are my top six reasons why flattening your belly is going to make your life better.

Reason 1: A Flat Belly Will Help You Live Longer

STUDY AFTER STUDY shows that the people with the largest waist sizes have the most risk of life-threatening disease. The evidence couldn't be more convincing. According to the National Institutes of Health, a waistline larger than 35 inches for women signals significant risk of heart disease and diabetes. One study in the *International Journal of Obesity* found that women should strive for waist sizes less than 31.5—because as your waist grows larger, so does your risk of heart disease. Now the real scary part: Federal health surveys show that over the past four decades the average American woman's waist size has grown from 30 inches to 37 inches—meaning she is at an increased risk for heart disease, stroke, and cancer. A study of 44,000 US women by National Institutes of Health and Harvard Medical School researchers published in 2008 found that abdominal obesity doubled women's odds of dying from cardiovascular disease compared with women whose waistlines were smaller than 28 inches.

Of course, finding your abs doesn't guarantee you a get-out-of-the-hospital-free card, but studies show that by developing a strong abdominal section, you'll reduce body fat and significantly cut the risk factors associated with many diseases, not just heart disease. For example, that same Harvard study found that women with the largest waists had a 63 perent greater risk of dying of cancer than women who were the most trim. The World Health Organization estimates that up to one-third of cancers of the colon, kidney, and digestive tract are caused by being overweight and inactive. A University of Minnesota study that tracked 22,000 women over 7 years found that overweight women who lost 20 or more pounds cut their risk of breast cancer by 19 percent. And having an excess of belly fat is especially dangerous. See, cancer is caused by mutations that occur in cells as they divide. Fat tissue in your abdomen spurs your body to produce hormones that prompt your cells to divide. More cell division means more opportunities for cell mutations, which means more cancer risk.

A lean waistline also heads off another of our most pressing health problems—diabetes. It is estimated that 23 million Americans now have type 2 diabetes, and one quarter of them don't even know it. In addition, 57 million more Americans may have pre-diabetes. Fat, especially belly fat, bears the blame. There's a misconception that diabetes comes only from eating too much refined sugar, like the kind in chocolate and ice cream. But people develop diabetes after years of eating high-carbohydrate foods that are easily converted into sugar—foods like white bread, pasta, and mashed potatoes. Scarfing down a basket of bread and a bowl of pasta can do the same thing to your body that a carton of ice cream does: flood it with sugar calories. The calories you can't burn are what convert into fat cells that pad your gut and leave you with a disease that, if untreated, can lead to blindness, heart attacks, strokes, amputation, and death. And that, my friend, can really ruin your day. But you can control a lot of this; a study tracking 1,400 diabetic people for 9 years found that just trying to lose weight could cut diabetes-related death risk by up to 30 percent.

Upper-body obesity is also the most significant risk factor for obstructive sleep apnea, a condition in which the soft tissue in the back of your throat collapses during sleep, blocking your airway. When that happens, your brain signals you to wake up and start breathing again. As you nod off once more, the same thing happens, and it can continue hundreds of times during the night—making you chronically groggy and unable to get the rest your body needs. Fat's role is that it can impede muscles that inflate and ventilate the lungs, forcing you to work harder to get enough air.

Being overweight also puts you at risk for a lot of other conditions that rob you of a good night's rest, including gastroesophageal reflux and asthma. A 3-year French study of 67,229 women found that being overweight doubled the risk of asthma, and women who gained about 20 pounds from the time they started menstruating to the time they reached adulthood had a 66 percent higher risk. All of this can create an ugly cycle: Abdominal fat leads to poor sleep. Poor sleep means you drag through your day. Sluggish and tired, your body craves some quick energy, so you snack on some high-calorie junk food. That extra junk food leads to more abdominal fat, which leads to . . . well, you get the picture.

I could fill this whole book with evidence, but I'm going to boil it down to one sentence: A smaller waist equals fewer health risks.

Reason 2: A Flat Belly Will Improve Your Sex Life

WOMEN CLAIM THE greatest sex organ is the brain; men say it's approximately 3 feet due south. So let's say we split the geographic difference and focus on what's really central to a good sex life.

For one, strong abdominal and lower-back muscles give you stamina and strength to try new positions (or stay steady in old ones), so that sex is as pleasurable as it should be. But even more important, a smaller waistline means that women will be better equipped in another important area—bloodflow.

Artery-clogging cheeseburgers don't discriminate, so when you're overweight, the gunk that gums up the blood vessels leading to your heart and brain also gums up the vessels that lead to your genitals. Plaque forms on the inside of your arteries, narrowing the passageways that blood must follow—meaning that blood has trouble making it to the pelvic area. Decreased flow of blood in the pelvic area in women can lead to decreased lubrication, sensitivity, and sexual pleasure.

At least one study of more than 200 women showed that by increasing bloodflow to the genital area of women, you could increase lubrication, sensitivity, arousal, and sensation to the area. Other research shows that exercise can improve libido. In the study, women who pedaled a stationary cycle for 20 minutes before watching an erotic video experienced a greater level of sexual arousal than women who didn't exercise before watching. Both studies, while preliminary, suggest that athletic pipes can play a role in sexual satisfaction.

Reason 3: A Flat Belly Will Keep You Safe from Harm

IN SCHOOL, YOU were taught the story of Mrs. O'Leary's cow and how, with one awkward misstep, the lumbering bovine knocked over an oil lamp that started the Great Chicago Fire and burned much of that toddlin' town to the ground. That tragedy happened at a time when most urban housing was still built with wood. Today, such a disaster is unthinkable—and not just because we don't let cows into the living room anymore. It's unthinkable because the infrastructure of today's cities is built with steel—steel that stands up to fire, earthquakes, and hurricanes.

Think of your midsection as your body's infrastructure. You don't want a core made of dry, brittle wood or straw. You want one made of solid steel, one that will give you a layer of protection that belly fat never could.

Consider a US Army study that linked powerful abdominal muscles to injury prevention. After giving 120 artillery soldiers the standard army fitness test of situps, pushups, and a 2-mile run, researchers tracked their lower-body injuries (such as lower-back pain and Achilles tendinitis) during a year of field training. The 29 soldiers who cranked out the most situps (73 in 2 minutes) were five times less likely to suffer lower-body injuries than the 31 who barely notched 50. But that's not the most striking element. Those who performed well in the pushups and 2-mile run enjoyed no such protection—suggesting that upper-body strength and cardiovascular endurance had little effect on keeping bodies sound. It was abdominal strength that offered the protection. Unlike any other muscles in your body, a strong core affects the functioning of the entire body. Whether you ski, do yard work, or carry the kids away from the candy aisle, your abs are the most essential muscles for keeping you from injury. The stronger they are, the stronger—and safer—you are.

Reason 4: A Flat Belly Will Strengthen Your Back

I HAD A friend who threw out his back maybe two or three times a year. He always did it in the simplest way—sleeping a little awkwardly or getting out of a chair too quickly. One time, he pulled it out reaching into the backseat of his car to get something his young daughter had dropped. The pain once stabbed him so badly that he collapsed to the ground while he was standing at a urinal. (Go ahead. Imagine that.) His problem wasn't that he had a bad back; it was that he had weak abs. If he had trained them regularly, he could've kept himself from being one of the millions of people who suffer from back pain every year. And yes, he started the Abs Diet Workout, and within weeks his back pain virtually disappeared.

ABS DIET SUCCESS STORY

"I found my inner athlete"

Name: Rebecca Carr

Age: 29

Height: 5'1½"

Starting Weight: 148

Current Weight: 118

Starting Waist Size: 32¾"

Current Waist Size: 26½"

Starting Dress Size: 10

Current Dress Size: 4

Rebecca Carr always felt that she was a little bit over a healthy weight.

"Growing up, I saw people who were into fitness and health and eating right, and I always thought that they were doing something right in life. I said, 'Hey, that's how I want to live.' I always wanted to be that person," she says.

One morning, Carr and her husband were watching TV and heard the Abs Diet mentioned on the morning news.

"Something just clicked in my head," she says. "It's what I believe in and it matches who I am, and it made sense. I bought the only copy of the book that was on the shelf at Borders and read it cover to cover."

Because most back pain is related to weak muscles in your trunk, maintaining a strong midsection can help resolve many back issues. The muscles that crisscross your midsection don't function in isolation; they weave through your torso like a spiderweb, even attaching to your spine. When your abdominal muscles are weak, the muscles in your butt (your glutes) and along the backs of your legs (your hamstrings) have to compensate for the work your abs should be doing. The effect, besides promoting bad company morale for the muscles picking up the slack, is that it destabilizes the spine and eventually leads to back pain and strain—or even more serious back problems.

Reason 5: A Flat Belly Will Help You Win

IF YOU RUN, bike, play naked Twister, or do any sport that requires movement, your essential muscle group isn't your legs or arms. It's your core—the muscles in your torso and hips. Developing core strength gives you power to perform.

Carr made adjustments to her diet, limiting her desserts and fried foods to the point where the onetime dessertaholic doesn't even miss them. (The weekly cheat meal that the Abs Diet allows keeps her in check: "If I want a burger and fries, I tell myself I can have it on the weekend if I want, but by the time the weekend comes, my interest is gone.")

Carr is never hungry, and she packs her daily meals the night before to help her manage eating during stressful days. Besides having improved skin and energy levels, Carr has also been inspired to push herself deeper into the world of fitness—she has completed 5-K and 10-K races, and now she's training for a half-marathon. "At 29 years old, I found my inner athlete," she says.

Now Carr's parents tell her that she's a different person—how motivating she is that she has such a healthy outlook. Carr's husband and father have both lost weight on the Abs Diet, having been motivated by her success.

"It doesn't feel like a diet," she says. "It feels like living."

It fortifies the muscles around your whole midsection and trains them to provide the right amount of support when you need it. So if you're weak off the serve, strong abs will improve it. If you also play sports where you run a lot, whether it's tennis or tag, abs can improve your game tremendously. That's because speed is really about accelerating and decelerating. How fast can you go from a stopped position at one baseline to stopping at the other baseline? Your legs don't control that; your abs do. When researchers studied which muscles were the first to engage in these types of sports movements, they found that the abs fired first. The stronger they are, the faster you'll get to the ball.

Reason 6: A Flat Belly Will Limit Your Aches and Pains

AS YOU AGE, it's common to experience some joint pain—most likely in your knees and hips, but maybe around your feet and ankles, too. The source of that pain might not be weak joints; it might be weak abs—especially if you do any

|||||||||||||||||||||||||||||||||||||||||||||||||||||||||||||||||||||||||||||||||||||||||||||||||||||||||||||||||||||

Abs Diet FAQs

How much weight will I lose on the New Abs Diet for Women?

I can't give you a firm number, because people's bodies have more variables than a calculus textbook. I can tell you that some people who have used the Abs Diet lost 25 pounds in 6 weeks. That doesn't necessarily mean that you will, but it means that you might or that you could. Much of your success depends on so many factors—including your intensity of exercise and your starting weight. But we've seen a lot of people who've lost somewhere between 10 and 15 pounds in the first 6 weeks while also gaining a few pounds of muscle, which helps them keep burning fat after that initial 6-week surge.

What percentage of body fat do you have to get to so that you can see your abs?

Finding your abs might feel as daunting as digging through sand to find a buried treasure. But if you dig diligently enough—and by that I mean burning off that extra, unwanted flab—you will find the treasure. As far as the specific body-fat percentage, it varies. I've seen both men and women with body-fat percentages in the teens with defined stomach muscles. The good news is that if you're exercising regularly, then at least 80 percent of every pound you lose will be fat.

kind of exercise, from serious tennis playing to walking every morning. When you're doing any type of athletic activity, your abdominal muscles help stabilize your body during start-and-stop movements, like changing direction on the tennis court or in kickboxing class. If you have weak abdominal muscles, your joints absorb all the force from those movements. It's kind of like trampoline physics. Jump in the center, and the mat will absorb your weight and bounce you back in the air. Jump toward the side of the trampoline, where the mat meets the frame, and you'll bust the springs. Your body is sort of like a trampoline, with your abs as the center of the mat and your joints as the supports that hold the mat to the frame. If your abs are strong enough to absorb some shock, you'll function well. If they're not, the force puts far more pressure on your joints than they were built to withstand.

Similar protection benefits extend to people who aren't athletes, too. One Dutch study of nearly 6,000 people found that those with larger waist sizes were more likely to have heel pain and develop carpal tunnel syndrome, a painful hand and wrist condition. One study even found that 70 percent of people with carpal tunnel syndrome were either overweight or obese.

• • •

These are all great reasons to pursue the Abs Diet. But the best reason is this: The program is an easy, sacrifice-free plan that will let you eat the foods you want and keep you looking and feeling better day after day. It's designed to help you lose weight in the easiest possible ways: by recalibrating your body's internal fat-burning furnace; by focusing on the foods that trigger your body to start shedding flab; and by rebuilding you into a lean, mean, fat-burning machine.

THE ABS DIET START-UP KIT

THIS SIMPLE SHOPPING LIST will give you everything you need to dive right into the New Abs Diet and the Abs Diet Workout.

BUY ONCE

Blender	Ground flaxseed, 1 pint	Multivitamins, such as Centrum, 1 jar

BASIC SHOPPING LIST—THE ABS DIET POWER 12 AND RELATED FOODS

Almonds, slivered or whole

Beans of choice

Spinach, fresh or frozen

Dairy (fat-free or low-fat milk and vanilla yogurt)

Instant oatmeal (unsweetened, unflavored)

Eggs

Turkey, sliced

Peanut butter, all-natural (no added sugar)

Olive oil

Whole-grain breads and cereals

Extra-protein (whey) powder, vanilla and chocolate, 1-quart containers

Raspberries, fresh and frozen

Plus:

Black beans

Blueberries, frozen

Canned tuna

Cannellini beans

Chicken breast

Craisins (dried, sweetened cranberries)

Garbanzo beans

Grapefruit

Green vegetables of choice

Italian salad greens

Lean ground beef

Long-grain rice

Mixed greens

Pecans

Pine nuts

Roasted cashews and peanuts, unsalted

Shrimp, frozen

Strawberries, fresh or frozen

Trout, smoked salmon, or other lean fish of choice

Whole-wheat pasta

SHOPPING LIST–INGREDIENTS FOR RECIPES

(SEE RECIPES FOR INDIVIDUAL AMOUNTS)

Avocado

Baby carrots

Balsamic and red wine vinegars

Bananas

Barbecue sauce

Basil

Beef jerky

Brown rice

Canadian bacon

Canned chicken stock

Canned mandarin orange slices

Canned peeled tomatoes

Canned pumpkin

Cantaloupe

Carnation Instant Breakfast packets

Cayenne pepper

Celery

Chili powder

Chives

Chocolate syrup

Cilantro

Cinnamon

Corn, frozen

Cornmeal

Cucumber

Curry powder

Dijon mustard

Dried chili mix

Fat-free mayonnaise

Flat bread

Flour

French baguette

French green beans

Fresh ginger

Garlic

Green and red bell peppers

Ground buffalo

Guacamole

Housin sauce

Honey

Honeydew melon

Honey-wheat English muffins

Instant grits

Italian-seasoned bread crumbs

Italian seasoning

Jalapeño peppers

Ketchup

Lean sirloin steak

Lean sliced roast beef

Lemons and limes

Lemon juice concentrate, frozen

Low-fat balsamic vinaigrette, ranch, and Thousand Island salad dressings

Low-fat ice cream (vanilla and butter pecan)

Low-fat Italian salad dressing packet

Maple syrup

Mexican-style tomatoes

Mint, fresh or dried

Mushrooms

Navy beans

Onions, green, red, and white

Onion soup mix

Orange juice

Oranges

Oregano

Paprika

Parsley

Peanut oil

Pork chops, boneless

Portobello mushrooms

Prosciutto

Red pepper flakes

Reduced-fat cheese (American, blue cheese, Cheddar, cottage, cream, feta, mozzarella, ricotta, Swiss)

Raisin bread

Raisins

Red and Granny Smith apples

Reduced-sodium soy sauce

Roasted red peppers

Romaine lettuce

Rosemary

Rye bread

Salsa

Saltine crackers or bread crumbs

Sauerkraut

Spaghetti sauce

Stir-fry sauce

Steel-cut oats

Sweet corn

Tabasco sauce

Tomatoes

Tomato sauce

Tortilla chips

Trans fat–free margarine

Turkey bacon

Turkey sausage

Watermelon

Whole-wheat pitas

Whole-wheat toaster waffles

Whole-wheat tortillas

Worcestershire sauce

FOR AT-HOME EXERCISE

(A GYM SHOULD HAVE ALL NECESSARY EQUIPMENT)

Exercise mat
(optional)

Flat bench
(optional but
recommended)

One or two pairs
of medium-weight
dumbbells (5 to
25 pounds for
someone with some
experience lifting
weights; lighter for
beginners)

Running shoes

Swiss ball (optional
but recommended)

Exercise bands for
resistance training
while traveling or
at home

Chapter 2

EAT THIS, WEIGH LESS
Why The Abs Diet Works When Others Fail

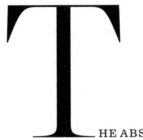

THE ABS DIET IS A SIMPLE plan built around 12 nutrient-packed foods that, when moved to the head of your dietary table, will give you all the vitamins, minerals, and fiber you need for optimum health while triggering lean muscle growth and firing up your body's natural fat burners. (Tell me this isn't a meal plan you can stick to!)

A lmonds and other nuts

B eans and legumes

S pinach and other green vegetables

D airy (fat-free or low-fat milk, yogurt, cheese)

I nstant oatmeal (unsweetened, unflavored)

E ggs

T urkey and other lean meats

P eanut butter

O live oil

W hole-grain breads and cereals

E xtra-protein (whey) powder

R aspberries and other berries

I've chosen these foods both for their nutritional content and their simplicity. That's why I based the Abs Diet on common foods that are easy to prepare and enjoy. The way I see it, most other diet plans are too complicated and invite failure in three major ways.

1. They reduce calories too severely. With a strict—or drastic—calorie reduction, you may lose weight at first, but you're left hungry. When you're hungry, you've increased the chances that you'll gorge at some point during the day. When you gorge, you feel as if you failed, then feel guilty for failing, then drop off the plan and resume your chocolate-for-breakfast habits. With the Abs Diet, however, you'll never go hungry—in fact, you'll find yourself eating much more often than you do now: six times a day!

2. They restrict too many foods. It would be easy to build a plan that didn't include pasta, pizza, or savory bruschetta. But if I did that,

---

ABS DIET SUCCESS STORY

"You're getting what women die for"

Name: Rhonda Hauser

Age: 38

Height: 5'8"

Weight: 140ish

Starting Body: Soft

Current Body: Strong

Built with a tall, lanky runner's body, Rhonda Hauser has never been one to care much about scales or taking measurements of herself. But she has been in and out of gyms for years, she's had a couple trainers, and she's gone to nutritionists because she cares about her body. But she also had a problem: Turns out she was overtraining and undereating (mostly eating kashi cereal and protein shakes). She wasn't overweight, but she didn't have the body she wanted.

"I saw the Abs Diet and thought it was really targeted for me," she says. "It reminded me that you have to eat, and you need foods with protein to build muscle, the internal fat burner."

you'd ditch the plan the first time you drove past your favorite Italian restaurant. Even though changing your eating habits is a fundamental part of this program, I think there's a greater chance you'll stick to the plan if you don't have to give up everything you like. It's normal to have steaks off the grill, Mom's pie at the holidays, a glass of wine or beer after work. If you deprive yourself of every food that tastes good, there's not much incentive for even the most motivated person to stick to the plan for longer than a few weeks. The Abs Diet is about eating the foods you enjoy—and indulging yourself when need be.

3. They don't take into account lifestyle. If we all had a chef to prepare our meals—or even more than a few minutes to do it ourselves—losing weight would be much simpler. But when was the last time you had 2 hours to prepare a meal? We're all busy. We eat in restaurants. We order in. We hit drive-throughs. We hustle food on the table to satisfy the needs of our families and to save as much energy as possible. Yes, we wish we

---

Hauser integrated more Power-foods into her diet and exchanged her mostly running regimen for the Abs Diet circuit workouts.

"When I started doing circuits, my body took on its own transformation," says Hauser, who got more definition in her arms and shoulders. "After a couple of weeks, people in the gym were looking at me and asking if I was training for an Ironman. I started feeling stronger, and my muscles were developing."

After 6 weeks, Hauser says, her pants started to feel a little weird. She hoped that she wasn't gaining weight from doing the exercises, so she asked her girlfriends if they could tell what was going on. "My glutes started to lift up and tighten.

My friends said, 'You're getting what women die for.' I call it the hubba heinie—a little round rump roast."

While Hauser still doesn't use a scale, she knows that her body has experienced a major change.

"The cool thing about it is that it gives me direction, and it's something I believe in," Hauser says. "Anything you believe in and consistently do is going to get you results. I carry this book around with me like it's my bible."

had time to tally fat-gram totals; measure every ounce of food; or prepare elaborate, good-for-you dishes. But the reality is that most of us won't, no matter how much weight we need to lose. We have commitments to jobs and families, and we spend so much time doing everything from commuting to paying the bills and taking care of the kids that a mango-shrimp masterpiece hardly tops the priority list. The Abs Diet is what you need: a low-maintenance program with low-maintenance foods and even lower-maintenance recipes.

For these reasons, many of today's most popular diets offer only short-term weight loss and long-term weight gain.

As I said in the introduction to this book, most diets are about losing—and Americans don't like to be losers. The New Abs Diet for Women is about gaining. The Abs Diet is based on the simple notion that your body is a living, breathing, calorie-burning machine and that by keeping your body's fat furnace constantly stoked with lots and lots of the right foods—and this is important—at the right time, you can teach it to start burning off your belly in no time. In fact, this diet can help you burn up to 12 pounds of fat—from your belly first—in 2 weeks or less. And just look at what you'll gain in return.

You'll gain meals. Americans have huge appetites. We hunger for success, we hunger for freedom, and yeah, we hunger for food. Traditional calorie- or food-restricting diets run counter to this uniquely American appetite. They leave us hungry, miserable, and one Twinkie away from a total couch collapse. But not the Abs Diet. You will eat on this program—and eat often. In fact, you'll be refueling constantly, and with every delicious meal or snack, you'll be stoking your body's natural fat burners. Imagine that: Every time you eat, you help your body lose weight and turn flab into abs.

You'll gain some tone. With the Abs Diet and the Abs Diet Workout, eating the right foods means you'll be growing more muscle. With added muscle, you'll lose more fat. This program converts the food you eat into muscle. The more lean muscle mass you have, the more energy it takes to fuel it—meaning that calories go toward sustaining your muscles rather than being converted to fat. In fact, research shows that adding lean muscle mass acts as a built-in fat burner. Again, for every pound of muscle you gain, your resting metabolic rate goes up as much as 50 calories a day. The strength-training component can put several pounds of muscle onto your body. You won't beef up like a bodybuilder, but you will build enough muscle to shrink and tighten your belly—and, depending on your starting point, show off your abs. When you add exercise into the mix, you can think of it as a simple equation.

MORE FOOD + MORE MUSCLE = LESS FLAB

Now, consider the alternative.

LESS FOOD + LESS MUSCLE = MORE FLAB

Isn't it incredible that most diets focus on the "less food" equation? And isn't it time we changed that? (Sure, some studies have shown that you'll live longer on a superrestrictive diet of less than 1,400 calories a day. But given how such a plan would make you feel, you probably wouldn't want to.)

You'll gain freedom. Most diets deprive you of something—whether it's carbs, fat, or fun. (Can I have a blue-cheese bacon burger, hold the bun? No thanks.) In this plan, you will not feel deprived. You'll stay full. You'll eat crunchy food. You'll eat sweet food. You'll eat protein, carbs, and fat. In fact, there's even one meal during the week when you can eat anything you want. Anything. During the bulk of the week, you'll focus on foods that will charge your metabolism and control your temptations, but you'll also have the freedom and flexibility to stray just enough to keep you satisfied without ruining all the work you've already put in.

You'll gain time. On some diets, it seems like it would take less time to raise a farm of chickens and wait for the eggs to drop than it would take to plan and cook the recipes they tout. On this diet, all of the meals and recipes are low maintenance. For planning purposes, all I want you to do is take this program 2 days at a time. Because mindless noshing is the nation's number-one diet buster, your best defense is to plot out a simple strategy for how and what you're going to eat each day. Every night, take 5 minutes to sketch out what and when you'll eat the next day, and you'll have deflated temptation and gained control. After reading the principles, you'll see that the Abs Diet establishes a new paradigm for weight control. Simply:

MORE FOOD + MORE MUSCLE = LESS FLAB

Chapter 3

BURN FAT DAY AND NIGHT

How Metabolism Shapes Your Body—
And How You Can Change Yours

I N CHAPTER 2, I DISCUSSED
how most popular diets are designed to offer only short-term weight loss and
how following these programs sets you up not only to regain the weight you
initially shed but also to actually gain even more fat in the long run. Most diets,
in fact, are not long-term fat-loss plans but long-term fat-gain plans. The Abs
Diet for Women is different: It's a program that helps you rev up your body's
natural fat burners and keep them revved for life.

As harmful as most diet crazes may be, diets alone aren't to blame for the
obesity epidemic in America. In fact, there's plenty of blame to go around: fast
food, funnel cakes, stress, sedentary lifestyles, supersizing, all-you-can-eat
buffets, the demise of physical education classes, free refills, couches, movie
theater popcorn, you name it. We're a society of overeaters who often hold desk
jobs and would lobby to make the Bloomin' Onion its own food group. But in
the battle of weight control, these are the easy targets. Instead, I'd argue, one
of the reasons we keep getting fatter is that we put our faith in two things that
are supposed to help us lose weight. These weight loss "double agents" reap

praise for their contributions to good health, but they've also done their part in skewing the way we think about weight loss. The two culprits I blame for our obesity epidemic: nutritional labels and exercise machines.

Is Calorie Counting Right for You?

BEFORE YOU BUST a button, hear me out. Labels and machines both have their appropriate uses (the former for the simple knowledge of the vitamins, minerals, and ingredients in your food; the latter for getting people off their duffs and exercising). My beef with labels and machines is not what they do per se but the myth they perpetuate. Through their function, they feed into a way of thinking about weight loss that actually makes it harder to control weight. They've turned us into a community of heavies who worship at the altar of one seemingly omnipotent number: the calorie.

With every food you eat and with every workout you finish, you look at how many calories come in and how many calories go out. It's the turnstile theory of weight loss: If you exercise away more than you take in, then you'll lose weight. Experts tell us that a pound of fat contains roughly 3,500 calories, so if you simply delete 500 calories from your daily meals, increase your daily exercise by 500 calories, or some combination thereof, you'll lose a pound of fat a week. That sounds great in theory, but in real life, the whole concept of calorie management is more likely to make you lose heart than lose weight. You hump it on the stairclimber for 30 minutes and sweat like a guest on *The O'Reilly Factor.* When you see the final readout—"Workout Completed; 300 Calories Burned!"—you feel like you've just chipped away at your belly and gotten closer to your goal. That is, until you reach for a nighttime snack and see that a serving and a half of raisin bran also equals 300 calories. What took 30 minutes to burn takes 30 seconds to dust off during *Desperate Housewives.* It's a psychological diet killer.

Of course, there's nothing wrong with using nutritional labels to track what you eat or as a deterrent to stay away from high-calorie foods in the first place. In fact, many women feel like they need calorie counting to help them stay within optimal daily targets, and that's okay—as long as you keep calories in perspective. It's better to focus on what's happening inside your body during the rest of your day—when you're working, sleeping, making love, or just sitting still right now reading this book. Right this very instant, your body is either gaining fat or losing fat. The Abs Diet will train your body to lose fat while you're sitting still because the Abs Diet focuses on something other diet plans miss: your metabolism.

What Is "Metabolism"?

METABOLISM IS THE rate at which your body burns its way through calories just to keep itself alive—to keep your heart beating, your lungs breathing, your blood pumping, and your mind fantasizing about the Caribbean while crunching year-end accounting figures or telling Timmy to go to a time-out. Your body is burning calories all the time, even while you're reading this sentence. The average woman burns about 10 calories per pound of body weight every day.

ABS DIET SUCCESS STORY

"I Needed Something That Was Easy"

Name: Linda Toomey

Age: 35

Height: 5'4"

Starting weight: 145

6 weeks later: 129

When Linda Toomey had her fourth baby, she knew that she had to get the weight off. She had kept 20 pounds on from her third baby and wanted to act quickly because she knew the longer she waited, the harder it would be. At 145 pounds and with four children under the age of 6, she knew that her own health—and belly—might take a backseat to everything else going on in her life. "I'm the queen of excuses," she says.

Toomey also knew that she needed as much energy as possible—especially considering she wasn't getting a full night's sleep anyway, caring for a newborn.

"At night, I expected to be tired," she says. "But I was tired 2 hours after I woke up."

There are three main types of calorie burn that happen throughout your day. Understand how they work, and you'll understand exactly why the Abs Diet is going to turn your body into a fat-burning machine.

Calorie burn #1: The thermic effect of eating. Between 10 and 30 percent of the calories you burn each day get burned by the simple act of digesting your food. Now that's pretty cool—satisfying your food cravings actually makes you burn away calories. But not all foods are created equal: Your body uses more calories to digest protein (about 25 calories burned for every 100 calories consumed) than it does to digest fats and carbohydrates (10 to 15 calories burned for every 100 calories consumed). That's why the Abs Diet concentrates on lean, healthy proteins. Eat more of them in a sensible way, and you'll burn more calories.

Calorie burn #2: Exercise and movement. Another 10 to 15 percent of your calorie burn comes from moving your muscles, whether you're pressing

Toomey's goals: Get her body back, have more energy, and strengthen her back to be able to meet the demands of carrying children.

"I tried other diets, but being so crazy and busy, I didn't have a lot of time for exercise or food preparation. I needed something that was easy and fast to prepare," Toomey says.

She found it in the Abs Diet.

"It's not really a diet," she says. "It's a lifelong eating plan. I think knowing that you can eat carbs and don't have to resist cravings was one of the key factors. The eating plan was extremely easy to follow, and the whole family could enjoy the meals. I didn't have to prepare different foods for myself."

Toomey also included the 20-minute exercise plan and strengthened her abdominals and lower back to the point where she has no problem lifting her children.

In 6 weeks, she dropped 16 pounds and went from 36 percent body fat to 25. And she also went from a size 14 dress to size 6.

"I'm hoping it motivates a lot of women," Toomey says. "In the past, after I was pregnant, the waist was extremely hard for me. I might have lost inches from everywhere else, but the waist was my real difficult area. It's amazing how it progressed in a short time."

weights overhead, running to catch the bus, or just twiddling your thumbs. Simply turning the pages of this book will burn calories.

Calorie burn #3: Basal metabolism. This one's the biggie. Your basal, or resting, metabolism refers to the calories you're burning when you're doing nothing at all. Sleeping, watching TV, sitting through yet another mind-numbing presentation on corporate profit-and-loss statements—you're burning calories all the while. In fact, between 60 and 80 percent of your daily calories are burned up just doing nothing. That's because your body is constantly in motion: Your heart is beating, your lungs are breathing, and your cells are dividing all the time, even when you sleep.

Add up the percentages, and you'll see that the majority of your daily calorie burn comes from physiological functions that you don't even think about—the thermic effect of eating and your basal metabolism. While exercise is important, you need to realize that the calories you burn off during exercise aren't that important. Let me repeat that: Exercise is important, but the calories you burn off during exercise aren't important. That's why the exercise program we outline in the Abs Diet is designed to alter your basal metabolism, turning your downtime into fat-burning time. And it's why the food choices we outline for you are designed to maximize the number of calories you burn simply by eating and digesting. I want you to forget about the calories you're burning during those 30 minutes in the gym and concentrate on the calories you're burning the other 23½ hours a day.

In effect, the Abs Diet is going to change your body into a fat-frying dynamo by several means.

Changing the Way You Exercise

HAVE YOU EVER seen a gym at rush hour? Everyone hovers around the treadmills, elliptical trainers, and stationary bikes. Signs warn you of 20-minute maximums so that the next sweat seeker can have his or her turn. It seems like everyone wants a cardiovascular, aerobic workout. The more you sweat, the more calories you burn, the more weight you lose, right? In a way, yes, the headphone-and-Lycra set is right. Cardiovascular exercise—steady-state endurance exercises, like running, biking, and swimming—burns a lot of calories. In fact, it often burns more than other forms of exercise like strength training or trendier workouts like yoga or Pilates. But when it comes to weight control, aerobic exercise is more overrated than the fall TV lineup. Why? For one reason: Aerobic exercise builds little (if any) muscle, and muscle is the key component of a speedy metabolism. Muscle eats fat; again, add 1 pound of muscle, and your body burns up to an additional 50 calories a day just to keep that muscle alive. Add 6 pounds of muscle, and suddenly you're burning up to 300 more calories each day just by sitting still.

Here's the problem with low-intensity aerobic exercise. Just like a car can't run without gas or a kite can't fly without wind, a body can't function without food. It's the fuel that helps you run, lift, and have sex. Generally, during exercise, your body calls upon glycogen (the stored form of carbohydrate in muscles and the liver), fat, and in some cases protein. When you're doing low-intensity aerobic exercise like jogging, your body primarily uses fat and glycogen (carbohydrates) for fuel. When it continues at longer periods (20 minutes or more), your body drifts into depletion: You exhaust your first-tier energy sources (your glycogen stores), and your body hunts around for the easiest source of energy it can find—protein. Your body actually begins to eat up muscle tissue, converting the protein stored in your muscles into energy you need to keep going. Once your body reaches that plateau, it burns up 5 to 6 grams of protein for every 30 minutes of ongoing exercise. (That's roughly the amount of protein you'll find in a hard-cooked egg.) By burning protein, you're not only missing an opportunity to burn fat but also losing all-important and powerful muscle. So aerobic exercise actually decreases muscle mass. Decreased muscle mass ultimately slows down your metabolism, making it easier for you to gain weight.

Now here's an even more shocking fact: When early studies compared cardiovascular exercise with weight training, researchers learned that people who engaged in aerobic activities burned more calories during exercise than those who tossed around iron. You'd assume, then, that aerobic exercise was the way to go. But that's not the end of the story.

It turns out that while lifters didn't burn as many calories during their workouts as the folks who ran or biked, they burned far more calories over the course of the next several hours. This phenomenon is known as the afterburn—the additional calories your body burns off in the hours and days after a workout. When researchers looked at the metabolic increases after exercise, they found that the increased metabolic effect of aerobics lasted only 30 to 60 minutes. The effects of weight training lasted as long as 48 hours. That's 48 hours during which the body was burning additional fat. Over the long term, both groups lost weight, but those who practiced strength training lost only fat, while the runners and bikers lost muscle mass as well. The message: Aerobic exercise essentially burns only at the time of the workout. Strength training burns calories long after you leave the gym, while you sleep, and maybe all the way until your next workout. Plus, the extra muscle you build through strength training means that in the long term, your body keeps burning calories at rest just to keep that new muscle alive.

That raises a question. What aspect of strength training creates the long afterburn? Most likely, it's the process of muscle repair. Weight lifting causes your muscle tissues to break down and rebuild themselves at a higher rate than normal. (Muscles are always breaking down and rebuilding; strength training simply accelerates the process.) That breakdown and rebuilding takes a lot of energy and could be what accounts for the long period of calorie burning. In fact, a Finnish study found that protein synthesis (the process that builds bigger muscles) increases 21 percent 3 hours after a workout.

The good news is that you don't have to lift like a Russian shot-putter to see the results. A recent Ohio University study found that a short but hard workout had the same effect as longer workouts. Using a circuit of three exercises in a row for 31 minutes, the subjects were still burning more calories than normal 38 hours after the workout. (The Abs Diet Workout is designed along similar principles to mimic these results.)

As I said earlier, building muscle increases your metabolism so much that you burn up to 50 calories per day per pound of muscle you have. The more muscle you have, the easier it is for you to lose fat. That's why one of the components of the plan includes an exercise program that will help you add the muscle you need to burn fat and reshape your body. And it also points to one of the reasons why you should deemphasize cardiovascular, aerobic exercise if you want to lose fat: because it depletes your body's store of fat-burning muscle.

Now, before you start thinking I'm some sort of antiaerobics fanatic, let me clarify a few things: I run almost daily, and I've even completed the New York City Marathon. Aerobic exercise burns calories, helps control stress, and improves your cardiovascular fitness. It also helps lower blood pressure and improve your cholesterol profile. If your choice is aerobic exercise or no exercise, for Pete's sake, get out there and run. But when it comes to long-term weight management, I'll take gym iron over road rubber any day.

Changing the Way You Eat

FEW THINGS IN American society have failed more often than diets (with the exception of your office's copy machine). I think there's an explanation for the high failure rate. For one, many diets have revolved around low-fat menus. I'll discuss fat in a later chapter, but one of the problems with low-fat diets is that they can suppress the manufacturing of testosterone, the hormone that contributes to the growth of muscle and the burning of fat. When testosterone levels are low, your body stores fat like squirrels store nuts. Many diets also fail because they don't take advantage of the single most powerful nutrient for building muscle and increasing your metabolism: protein.

Protein—in proportion with foods from other groups—works in two primary ways. First, eating more protein cranks up the thermic effect of digestion by as much as one-third. Second, protein is also the nutrient that builds calorie-consuming muscle. In effect, you get a double burn—while you're digesting food and later as it helps build muscle. In the Abs Diet, you'll emphasize protein for these very reasons, but you'll also emphasize the most powerful sources of protein. A Danish study published in the *American Journal of Clinical Nutrition* took a group of people and gave them diets that were high in protein from either pork or soy. They found that people on the diet higher in animal protein burned 2 percent more calories during a 24-hour period than those on the soy protein diet, despite the fact that they ate slightly less food. That's 34 calories a day if you're eating a 1,700-calorie diet. In other words, if you want to burn calories, tenderloin is better than tofu.

Changing the Way You Think
About the Word Diet

HERE'S A TYPICAL diet scenario: You nibble on a piece of toast for breakfast and some baby carrots for lunch, and you figure that puts you well ahead

(continued on page 40)

What the Heck Is . . . High Blood Pressure?

You know high blood pressure is bad, but you probably have a little trouble getting your head around the whole concept of how "blood pressure" works. Can't we just let a little of the blood out and lower the pressure, you might wonder. If only it were so easy.

When most people think of blood pressure, they think in terms of a garden hose: too much pressure and the hose bursts, unless you open the valve. But that model is too simple. It helps instead to think of your circulatory system as more like the Erie Canal—a series of locks and gates that help move blood around to where it's needed. See, gravity works on your blood just like it works on the rest of your body: It wants to pull everything downward. So imagine yourself hopping out of bed tomorrow morning and standing up. Gravity wants to take all that blood that's distributed throughout your body and pull it down into your feet. You, on the other hand, would like that blood to pump to your brain, where it can help you figure out where the hell your keys are.

On cue, arteries in the lower body constrict while the heart dramatically increases output. The instant result: Blood pressure rises, and blood flows to the brain. Ahh, there they are—in the dog's water dish, right where you left them.

It's an ingenious system, but one that's incredibly easy to throw out of whack. When you pack on extra padding around your stomach, your heart pumps harder to force blood into all that new fatty tissue. When you nosh on potato chips and other high-sodium foods, your body retains water in order to dilute the excess sodium, increasing overall blood volume. When you line your arteries with plaque from too many fatty meals, pressure increases as the same amount of blood has to squeeze through newly narrowed vessels. When you let the pressures of the day haunt you into the night, your brain pumps out stress hormones that keep your body in a perpetual state of fight-or-flight anxiousness, also forcing your heart to pump harder. High-salt, high-fat diets and an excess of stress all combine to create a dangerous situation.

Much to the dismay of Quentin Tarantino fans, letting out some blood won't relieve the pressure. Your heart is still pumping, and your blood vessels are still dilating and contracting to make sure the blood goes where it's needed. When the pressure remains high for years on end, thin-walled vessels in the brain can burst under extreme pressure; brain cells die as a result in what's known as a hemorrhagic stroke. Or hypertension can cause plaque buildup in one of the brain's arteries, eventually cutting off blood-flow. (High blood pressure damages smooth artery walls, creating anchor points for plaque to latch on to.) Kidney failure or a heart attack can also follow from dangerous plaque accumulations.

Then there's the plain old wear and tear that high blood pressure causes on your ticker. Over time, the extra work brought on by high blood pressure causes the walls of the heart to stiffen and thicken. The heart becomes a less efficient pump, unable to push out as much blood as it takes in. Blood backs up, the heart gives out, and the coroner scribbles "congestive heart failure" on your chart.

Ideally, your blood pressure should be lower than 120/80. What do those numbers mean? The top number, called the systolic pressure, is the pressure generated when the heart beats. The bottom number is the diastolic pressure, the pressure on your blood vessels when the heart is resting between beats. Higher readings are broken out into three categories.

> ▶ **Prehypertensive: 120–139 systolic/80–89 diastolic.**
> Prehypertensives should start worrying now about their blood pressure, concentrating on diet and exercise tips like those found in the Abs Diet. You may not see the flashing lights in your mirror right now, but your radar detector just went off. Time to slow down.

> ▶ **Stage I hypertensive: 140–159 systolic/90–99 diastolic.**
> For people who fall in this range, drug therapy is usually recommended in addition to lifestyle changes. Your risk of heart attack or stroke is elevated, and you need to be under a doctor's care.

> ▶ **Stage II hypertensive: 160 or greater systolic/100 or greater diastolic.** Advanced drug therapy is often a must for people at this level, who face a serious risk of being maimed or killed by their condition.

So, two questions: Do you know what your blood pressure is? If not, are you freaked out enough by now to start taking care of it? Fortunately, the Abs Diet Powerfoods can help by cutting down on the bad fats in your diet and increasing the good ones—and by slashing away some of those extra pounds. So can the Abs Diet Workout, as well as a few stress-reduction techniques. (To find out how you can help manage your stress level, see Chapter 18) In the meantime, try attacking the problem with some of these simple tips.

Cut salt, slice bananas. A study published in a 2009 edition of the the *Archives of Internal Medicine* suggests that a combination of eating more potassium-rich foods

(continued)

What the Heck Is . . . High Blood Pressure? (cont.)

while reducing sodium intake is more effective at reducing blood pressure than doing any one of those strategies alone. The study at Loyola University showed that cardiovascular disease increased by 50 percent for participants with a high sodium-to-potassium ratio in their blood. Potassium helps sweep excess sodium from the circulatory system, causing the blood vessels to dilate. But only about 1 percent of women get adequate amounts of this mineral. Other good sources of potassium are sweet potatoes, spinach, raisins, papayas, lima beans, and tomatoes.

Make it a low-sodium V8. Make that two 5.5-ounce cans: 11 ounces of V8 contains nearly 1,240 milligrams (mg) of potassium. The tomato juice also contains lycopene and lutein, two phytochemicals that have their own blood pressure–lowering properties.

Cut out the cold cuts. One slice of ham contains 240 milligrams of sodium, more salt than you'll find on the outside of two pretzel rods. The point: Lose the lunchmeat, and lower your blood pressure. A recent study found that prehypertensive people who reduced their daily sodium consumption from 3,300 to 1,500 milligrams knocked nearly 6 points off their systolic blood pressure and close to 3 off their diastolic. If you want to have your hoagie and eat it, too, at least switch to the Boars Head line of low-sodium meats—ham, turkey, roast beef—and leave the pickle on your plate (833 milligrams of sodium). Another rule of thumb: If a food comes canned or jarred, it's probably a salt mine.

Go two rounds and out. Make the second drink of the night your last call for alcohol. In a landmark study published in the *New England Journal of Medicine,* researchers found that one or two drinks a day actually decreased blood pressure slightly. Three drinks or more a day, however, elevated blood pressure by an average of 10 points systolic and 4 diastolic. The type of alcohol doesn't matter. Heck, order a screwdriver: Orange juice is one of the best sources of blood pressure-lowering potassium.

Drink more tea. An American Heart Association study found that people who drank 2 cups of tea a day were 25 percent less likely to die of heart disease than those who rarely touched the stuff. The reason: Flavonoids in the tea not only improve blood vessels' ability to relax but also thin the blood, reducing clotting.

Top your toast. Black currant jelly is a good source of quercetin, an antioxidant that Finnish researchers believe may improve heart health by preventing the buildup of the free radicals that can damage arterial walls and allow plaque to penetrate.

Have a Mac(intosh) attack. People who frequently eat apples have a 20 percent lower risk of developing heart disease than those who eat apples less often.

Eat fresh berries. Raspberries, strawberries, and blueberries are all loaded with salicylic acid—the same heart-disease fighter found in aspirin.

Order the tuna. Omega-3 fats in tuna and other fish help strengthen heart muscle, lower blood pressure, prevent clotting, and reduce levels of potentially deadly inflammation in the body.

Squeeze a grapefruit. One grapefruit a day can reduce arterial narrowing by 46 percent, lower your bad cholesterol level by more than 10 percent, and help drop your blood pressure by more than 5 points.

Eat oatmeal, an Abs Diet Powerfood! In two large and long-term studies, people who ate whole-grain foods instead of refined carbs significantly lowered their risk of hypertension.

Buy calcium-fortified OJ. Increasing the calcium in your diet can lower your blood pressure. Get 1,200 mg of calcium daily. By drinking calcium-enriched orange juice, you'll derive a benefit from the vitamin C as well. According to research from England, people with the most vitamin C in their bloodstreams are 40 percent less likely to die of heart disease.

Snack on pumpkin seeds. One ounce of seeds contains 151 milligrams of magnesium, more than a third of your recommended daily intake. Magnesium deficiencies have been linked to most risk factors for heart disease, including high blood pressure, elevated cholesterol levels, and increased buildup of plaque in the arteries. Other great sources: halibut (170 milligrams in 7 ounces of fish), brown rice (1 cup, 84 milligrams), chickpeas (1 cup, 79 milligrams), cashews (1 ounce, 74 milligrams), and artichokes (one gives you 72 milligrams).

Change your oil. Researchers in India found that people who replaced the corn and vegetable oils in their kitchens with monounsaturated fats (olive oil or, in this case, sesame seed oil) lowered their blood pressure by more than 30 points in just 60 days without making any other changes in their diets.

Cut down on candy snacking and soda drinking. New research is finding that sugar can raise blood pressure. Try to consume no more than 6 teaspoons of sugar daily.

of the calorie-counting game. By dinner, though, you've got so many onion rings jammed into your mouth that you look like Dizzy Gillespie. If you're so restricted in what you can eat, you'll eventually act like a rebellious teen and break the rules. While most diets say "no" more than a toddler with a plate of spinach, the Abs Diet gives you options. Most diets are about restricting. This one is about fueling.

For years—or maybe for all your life—you've probably had one notion about what dieting needs to be. Restrict your foods, eat like a supermodel, sweat on the treadmill, and you'll lose fat. In reality, those could be the very reasons why you couldn't lose weight. It's why you gained back what you lost. It's the reason why your speedboat metabolism may have geared down to that of an anchored barge. It's why you don't see much progress when you try new weight loss programs. And it's why the only real recipe many diet plans offer is a recipe for pecan-encrusted failure. What the Abs Diet will do is reprogram your circuitry. You'll stop thinking about every calorie and start thinking about how best to burn calories. Once you master that, your body will be equipped with all the tools it needs to strip away fat—and show off your belly.

Chapter 4

HOW THE NEW ABS DIET WORKS

What Your Last Meal Is Doing to Your Body Right Now

I N THE CRUDEST FORM, the way in which food travels through your body seems simple. There's one way in and one way out, and anything left behind snowballs into a mound of fat on your stomach, over your hips, on the backs of your arms, around your thighs, or under your chin. In reality, the travel patterns of your breakfast, lunch, and dinner flow more like a Los Angeles interstate system than anything else. You've got the traffic jams (clogged arteries) and the occasional drive-by shootings (indigestion), but you also have a complex network of roads that shuttle nutrients to and from vital organs and tissues. Your ability to lose weight and gain a little muscle largely depends on how and when you fuel your body to work in that system.

In the previous chapter, I showed how the key to effective weight management is concentrating on your body's calorie burn—not on how effectively you burn calories while exercising but on how effectively you burn calories when you're not exercising. Additionally, I explained a little about how the foods you eat can affect your body's daily calorie burn. Before I explain the how-tos of the Abs Diet, you should know the most important substances and nutrients that affect the way your body processes food.

Protein: The Most Valuable Nutrient

IN JUST ABOUT every area of life, few things are as admired as versatility—a mom who can shoot a basketball as well as she can cook, a dad who can change the oil and make a mean marinara sauce, a corporate president who can also fix the computers, a quarterback who runs as well as he throws, a singer who can dance as well as she can lip-synch. In your body, protein is the most versatile player on your nutrient team. It comes in many forms and does so many things well—all without a multimillion-dollar contract.

▶ Protein builds the framework of your body, including muscles, organs, bones, and connective tissues.

▶ In the form of enzymes, it helps your body digest food.

▶ As a hormone, it tells your body when to use food as energy and when to store it as fat.

▶ It transports oxygen through your blood to your muscles and organs.

▶ As an antibody, it protects you from illness when viruses and bacteria attack.

So protein is critical for helping your body function at optimum levels. But we've made protein the foundation of the Abs Diet for four other crucial reasons.

1. It tastes good. Sliced smoked turkey. Roasted pork loin. Steamed lobster. Peanut butter. The Abs Diet is built around the foods you crave, so it's a program you're not going to have to stick to; it's a program you're going to want to stick to.

2. It burns calories even as you're indulging in it. Food contains energy in the form of chemical bonds, but your body can't use them in that form. Your body has to break down the food and extract energy from that chemical bond; that process of extracting energy itself requires energy, so your body's burning more calories to do it. That's the thermic effect of eating, as I explained in Chapter 3, and protein pushes the thermic effect into high gear. It takes almost two times more energy to break down protein than it does to break down carbohydrates. So when you feed your body a greater amount of protein, your body automatically burns more calories throughout the day. When Arizona State University researchers compared the benefits of a high-protein diet with those of a high-carbohydrate diet, they found that people who ate a high-protein diet burned more than twice as many calories in the hours after their meals as those eating predominantly carbs.

3. It keeps you feeling satisfied. Research has shown that if you base your meals around protein, you'll feel fuller faster. Consider one study in the *European Journal of Clinical Nutrition*. Subjects downed one type of four different kinds of shakes—60 percent protein, 60 percent carbohydrate, 60 percent fat, or a mixture with equal amounts of all three. Then they were offered lunch. The subjects who had either the high-protein or mixed- nutrient shakes ate the least for lunch. Their shakes contained the same number of calories, but the protein made them feel fuller and therefore they ate less at lunchtime.

4. It builds muscle and keeps your body burning fat all day. Remember, muscle burns fat. When you lift and lower weights, you create microscopic tears in your muscles. To repair the tears, protein acts like the Red Cross. Your body parachutes in new protein to assess the damage and repair the muscle. Proteins fortify the original cell structure by building new muscle fibers.

This whole process through which proteins make new muscle fibers after a workout can last anywhere from 24 to 48 hours. So if you lift weights 3 days a week—triggering proteins to rush in and repair your muscles—your body essentially stays in muscle-building, and thus fat-burning, mode every day.

As you know, protein comes in many forms—such as turkey, beef, fish, nuts, and tofu. You want to concentrate on the proteins that best help build your muscles. Research has shown that animal protein builds muscle better than soy or vegetable protein does. So poultry, fish, and lean cuts of beef or pork are better choices than tofu or other soy-based products (though they are viable options, if you're a vegetarian). If you're the kind of person who likes to count, you'll want to shoot for about 1 gram of protein per pound of body weight per day—that's roughly the amount of protein your body can use every day. For a 130-pound woman, that's 130 grams of protein a day, which would break down into something like this:

3 eggs (18 grams)

2 cups of 1 percent milk (16 grams)

1 cup of cottage cheese (28 grams)

2½ ounces of peanuts (16 grams)

8 ounces of chicken breast (54 grams)

Combine those four reasons—an easy and delicious eating plan, greater calorie burn, less calorie intake, and more fat-burning muscle—and you can easily see how a high-protein diet translates into weight loss. In a Danish study, researchers put 65 subjects on a 12 percent protein diet, a 25 percent protein diet, or no diet (the control group). In the first two groups, the same percentage of calories—about 30 percent—came from fat. While the low-protein dieters lost an average of more than 11 pounds, the high-protein subjects lost an average of 20 pounds and ate fewer calories than the low-protein group.

The more amazing statistic wasn't how much they lost but where they lost it: The high-protein dieters also lost twice as much abdominal fat. One reason may be that a high-protein diet helps your body control its levels of cortisol, a stress hormone that causes fat to converge in the abdominal region.

Fat: Underrated, Understand?

WHEN YOU THINK of fat, you probably think of foods that have a lot of fat—or people who do. After a few years with some extra pounds, the only thing you know about fat is that you're tired of it and want to get rid of it forever. But it's probably one of your body's most misunderstood dietary nutrients, stemming from a widely held but misguided belief that fat should take much of the blame for our obesity epidemic.

In the 1980s, the US government released nutritional guidelines that essentially said we should base our diets on potatoes, rice, cereal, and pasta and minimize the foods with a lot of fat and protein. That gave way to the idea that fat makes you fat. And that gave way to a new breed of diets that said if you limit the fat in what you eat, you'll limit the fat that exercises squatter's rights on your belly. But that line of thinking didn't hold out when researchers tried to find links between low-fat diets and obesity. In 1998, for example, two prominent obesity researchers estimated that if you took only 10 percent of your calories from fat, you'd lose 16 grams of fat a day—a loss of 50 pounds in a year. But when a Harvard epidemiologist, Walter Willett, tried to find evidence that this occurred, he couldn't find any link between people who lost weight and the fact that they were on a low-fat diet. In fact, in some studies lasting a year or more, groups of people showed weight gains on low-fat diets. Willett speculated that there was a mechanism responsible for this: When the body is on a low-fat diet for a long period, it stops losing weight.

Part of the reason our bodies rebel against low-fat diets is that we need fat. For instance, fat plays a vital role in the delivery of vitamins A, D, E, and K, nutrients stored in fatty tissue and the liver until your body needs them. Fat also helps produce testosterone, which helps trigger muscle growth. And fat, like protein, helps keep you satisfied and controls your appetite. In fact, if we've learned anything about weight loss over the past several years, it's that reducing your fat intake doesn't necessarily do a darn thing to decrease your body fat. One small study, for instance, compared a high-carbohydrate diet and a high-fat diet. The researchers found that the group with the high-fat diet experienced less muscle loss than the other group. The researchers theorized that muscle protein was being spared by the higher-fat diet because fatty acids, more so than carbs, were being harnessed and used for energy.

The truth is that reasonable amounts of fat can actually help you lose weight. In a study from the *International Journal of Obesity,* researchers at Boston's Brigham and Women's Hospital and Harvard Medical School put 101 overweight people on either a low-fat diet (fat was 20 percent of the total calories) or a moderate-fat diet (35 percent of calories) and followed them for 18 months. Both groups lost weight at first, but after a year and a half, the moderate-fat group had lost an average of 9 pounds per person, whereas the low-fat dieters had gained 6 pounds. The results suggest that a healthy amount of fat is a factor in keeping your weight under control.

Here's a primer on the fats in your life.

Trans fat: BAD. More and more, you're seeing trans fat listed on food labels. Though it's in more than 40,000 packaged foods, it's so bad for you that food manufacturers have fought for years to keep it off ingredient labels.

In 2003, the US Food and Drug Administration finally adopted regulations requiring manufacturers to include trans fat content on their packaging. The regulations have been phased in over the past few years. It still helps to be a smart food consumer in order to spot where the danger lies.

Trans fats were invented by grocery manufacturers in the 1950s as a way of appealing to our natural cravings for fatty foods. But there's nothing natural about trans fats. They're cholesterol-raising, heart-weakening, diabetes-causing, belly-building chemicals that, for the most part, didn't even exist until the middle of the last century, and some studies have linked them to an estimated 30,000 premature deaths in this country every year. In one Harvard study, researchers found that getting just 3 percent of your daily calories from trans fats increased your risk of heart disease by 50 percent. Three percent of your daily calories equals about 7 grams of trans fats; that's roughly the amount in a single order of fries. Americans eat an average of between 3 and 10 grams of trans fats every day.

To understand what trans fats are, picture a bottle of vegetable oil and a stick of margarine. At room temperature, the vegetable oil is a liquid, the margarine a solid. Now, if you baked cookies using vegetable oil, they'd be pretty greasy. And who would want to buy a cookie swimming in oil? So to create cookies—and cakes, nachos, chips, pies, muffins, doughnuts, waffles, and many, many other foods we consume daily—manufacturers heat the oil to very high temperatures and infuse it with hydrogen. That hydrogen bonds with the oil to create an entirely new form of fat—trans fat—that stays solid at room temperature. Vegetable oil becomes margarine. And now foods that might normally be healthy—but maybe not as tasty—become fat bombs.

Because these trans fats don't exist in nature, your body has a hell of a time processing them. Once consumed, trans fats are free to cause all sorts of mischief inside you. They raise the number of LDL (bad) cholesterol particles in your bloodstream and lower your HDL (good) cholesterol. They also raise blood levels of other lipoproteins; the more lipoproteins you have in your bloodstream, the greater your risk of heart disease. Increased consumption of trans fats has also been linked to increased risk of diabetes and cancer.

Yet trans fats are added to a shocking number of foods. They appear on food labels as partially hydrogenated oil—usually vegetable or palm oil. Go look in your pantry and freezer right now, and you won't believe how many foods include them. Crackers. Popcorn. Cookies. Fish sticks. Cheese spreads. Candy bars. Frozen waffles. Stuffing. Even foods you might assume are healthy—like bran muffins, cereals, and nondairy creamers—are often loaded with trans fats. And because they hide in foods that look like they're low in fat, such as Wheat Thins, these fats are making you unhealthy without your even knowing it.

Take control of your trans fat intake. Check the ingredient labels on all the packaged foods you buy, and if you see partially hydrogenated oil on the label, consider finding an alternative. Even foods that seem bad for you can have healthy versions: McCains shoestring french fries, Ruffles Natural reduced-fat chips, Wheatables reduced-fat crackers, and Dove dark chocolate bars are just a few of the "bad for you" snacks that are actually free of trans fats. And remember—the higher up on the ingredients list partially hydrogenated oil is, the worse the food is for you. You might not be able to avoid trans fats entirely, but you can choose foods with a minimal amount of the stuff.

The other way to avoid trans fats is to avoid ordering fried foods. Because trans fats spoil less easily than natural fats and are easier to ship and store, almost all fried commercial foods are now fried in trans fats rather than natural oils. Fish and chips, tortillas, fried chicken—all of them are packed with belly-building trans fats. Order food baked or broiled whenever possible. And avoid fast-food joints, where nearly every food option is loaded with trans fats; drive-through restaurants ought to come complete with drive-through cardiology clinics.

AVOID

Margarine

Fried foods

Commercially manufactured baked goods

Any food with partially hydrogenated oil on its list of ingredients

Saturated fat: BAD. Saturated fats are naturally occurring fats found in meat and dairy products. The problem with saturated fats is that when they enter your body, they tend to do the same thing they did when they were in a pig's or cow's body: Rather than be burned for energy, they're more likely to be stored as fat in your flanks, in your ribs, even—ugh—in your loins.

In fact, they seem to have more of a "storage effect" than other fats. A study from Johns Hopkins University suggests that the amount of saturated fat in your diet may be directly proportional to the amount of fat surrounding your abdominal muscles. Researchers analyzed the diets of 84 people and performed an MRI on each of them to measure fat. Those whose diets included the highest rates of saturated fat also had the most abdominal fat. Saturated fats also raise cholesterol levels, so they increase your risk for heart disease and some types of cancer.

I don't want you to eliminate saturated fats entirely; they're found in most animal products, and those food products are important to the Abs Diet for other reasons (the calcium in dairy products, the protein in meat). But I do want you to consume the low-fat and leaner versions of meat and dairy products. You want the nutritional benefit from one part of the food without high amounts of saturated fat.

AVOID

Fatty cuts of red meat

Whole-milk dairy products

Polyunsaturated fats: GOOD. There are two types of polyunsaturated fats: omega-3s and omega-6s. You've probably heard of omega-3 fatty acids. They're the fats found in fish, and a diet high in omega-3s has been shown to help protect the heart from cardiovascular disease. That's plenty enough reason to include seafood in your diet. But new evidence suggests that this type of fat can actually help you control your weight. In one study, subjects who took in 6 grams a day of fish oil supplements burned more fat during the course of a day than those who went without. Researchers suspect that a diet high in omega-3s actually alters the body's metabolism and spurs it to burn fat more efficiently.

Now, you can take fish oil supplements if you want, but you'll miss the muscle-building protein benefits of real fish. The fish with the highest levels of omega-3s are the fish you probably enjoy the most already—salmon and tuna, to name two. (To see where your favorite fish falls in the omega-3 sweepstakes, see the chart on page 50.) In addition to being packed with heart-healthy, fat-burning omega-3s, fish is also a great source of lean, muscle-building protein.

There's another amazing, secret Powerfood that bodybuilders know about but you may have never even heard of: flaxseed. Flax is a seldom-used grain that's loaded with omega-3s as well as cholesterol-busting fiber. You'll find flaxseed in most health food stores. Grab it! I keep ground flaxseed in the fridge, and I toss it on breakfast cereals, into smoothies, and on top of ice cream. It's got a mild nutty flavor you'll like. It crushes cholesterol with its omega-3s, it adds artery-scouring fiber to your diet, and it might just be your best weapon against fat.

Omega-6 fatty acids also help lower bad cholesterol and raise good cholesterol. They're found in vegetable oils, meat, eggs, and dairy products. They're so common to so many foods, in fact, that only those of you currently shipwrecked on deserted islands living off flotsam and jetsam need worry about not getting enough in your diet.

EAT MORE

Fish
Flaxseed

Monounsaturated fats: GOOD. Monounsaturated fats are found in nuts, olives, peanuts, avocados, and olive and canola oils. Like omega-3s, these fats help reduce cholesterol levels and protect against heart disease, but they also help you burn fat; in one study, researchers found that the body burns more fat in the 5 hours following a meal high in monos than after a meal rich in saturated fats.

Monounsaturated fats will not only lower your cholesterol and help you burn off your belly but also help you eat less. Penn State researchers found that people who ate mashed potatoes prepared with oil high in monounsaturated fats like olive oil felt fuller longer than when they ate taters cooked with polyunsaturated fats like vegetable oil.

Carbohydrates: A Bad Rap

WITH THE BEATINGS that carbohydrates have taken over the past few years, it's a wonder that bread isn't protected by the Endangered Species Act. Everywhere I look, I see people eating burgers without buns, ordering spaghetti and meatballs—hold the spaghetti—or bragging about their all-bacon-all-the-time diet. While it's clear that protein and fat have tremendous nutritional benefits, it's unfair—and unhealthy—to kick carbohydrates off the dietary island.

With more and more evidence showing that a high-carbohydrate diet helps promote fat storage (unless you run marathons), it's becoming more accepted that low-carbohydrate diets work in helping people control weight. A study in the journal *Metabolism* confirmed that very stance. Researchers at the University of Connecticut found that subjects who ate only 46 grams of carbohydrates a day—about 8 percent of calories—lost 7 pounds of fat and gained 2 pounds of muscle in 6 weeks. But you can make a major mistake by eliminating carbohydrates entirely. Many carbohydrates—like fruits, vegetables, whole grains, and beans—help protect you against cancer and other diseases, and some carbs contain nutrients like fiber, which helps you lose and control weight.

|||||||||||||||||||||||||||||||||||||||||||||||||||||||||||||||||||||||||||||||||||||||||||||||||||||||

Seafood with the Highest Omega-3 Content

All data are for 3-ounce servings (except for sardines, which is for 3³⁄₄ ounces). Aim for a total of 2.5 grams (g) of omega-3s per day.

TYPE OF FISH	OMEGA-3 CONTENT (G)	PREPARED
Shad	3.7	Baked
Sardines	2.4	Water-packed can
Mackerel	1.9	Broiled
Sablefish	1.9	Broiled
Salmon	1.6	Poached
Tuna	1.5	Grilled
Oysters	1.4	Boiled
Trout	1.2	Broiled
Shark	1.1	Grilled
Swordfish	1.1	Grilled
Tuna, light	0.24	Water-packed can

Traditionally, the confusion about carbohydrates has centered around finding ways to classify them and figuring out which ones are better for your body. It used to be that we thought of carbohydrates only by their molecular structure—either simple or complex. Simple indicates a carb with one or two sugar molecules—things like sucrose (table sugar), fructose (in fruit), and lactose (in dairy products). Complex carbohydrates are ones that include more than two sugar molecules—like pasta, rice, bread, and potatoes. The flaw is that you can't generalize and say a carbohydrate is good or bad for you based simply on its molecular structure. For example, an apple contains nutrients and helps keep you lean; sugar does not. Both are simple carbs, but they're hardly comparable in nutritional value.

Instead, the way to decide what carbohydrates are best for you stems from how your body reacts to the carbohydrates chemically. One of the tools that nutritionists use today is the glycemic index (GI). The GI assigns numbers to foods that indicate how quickly a food turns into glucose. High-GI foods—ones that are quickly digested and turned to glucose—are generally less nutritionally sound than low-GI choices.

Another term for glucose is "blood sugar." The presence of sugar in your blood causes your body to produce the hormone insulin. Insulin's job is to move the sugar you're not using for energy out of your bloodstream and store it in your body. Here's where the GI comes into effect: Foods with a high GI (like pasta, bread, white rice, and Snickers bars) are digested quickly, flooding your bloodstream with sugar. Insulin rushes in and says, "Whoa, what do I do with all of this?" Whatever glucose isn't immediately burned for energy quickly starts getting stored as fat. What's worse is that if you eat a carb with a high GI in combination with fat—bread with butter, for example—none of the fat you eat can be burned for energy either, because your bloodstream is so flooded with sugar. Insulin does such a good job of turning this new blood sugar into fat, in fact, that soon your blood sugar begins to drop, and you know what that means: You're hungry again.

If you eat a meal with a low GI (like a balanced dinner of chicken, high-fiber vegetables, and brown rice), the food is digested more slowly. Your blood sugar rises only incrementally, and that slow digestion means that glucose is available as energy for hours and hours. That means you have hours and hours to burn off the blood sugar. Insulin doesn't need to rush in and turn the sugar into fat; it can use the sugar slowly for other construction projects, like building and repairing muscle. Moreover, because your blood sugar levels stay even, you don't turn ravenously hungry just a few hours after eating. You build more muscle, store less fat, have more energy, and keep your appetite under control.

By the way, if all this talk about blood sugar and insulin reminds you of a certain health problem—diabetes—then you were obviously paying attention in health class. Continuing to flood your bloodstream with high levels of sugar, followed by high levels of insulin, eventually trains your body to become less efficient at processing these blood sugars. That's called insulin resistance, which is another term for diabetes. It is a terrible, terrible disease—and it is also highly preventable. In a Harvard study, those who ate foods with the lowest GIs, such as whole-wheat bread, were 37 percent less likely to develop diabetes than those who ate high-GI foods, such as white rice. For more information on battling diabetes, see our Health Bulletin on page 70.

|||||||||||||||||||||||||||||||||||||||||||||||||||||||||||||||||||||||||||||||||||||||||||||||||||||||||||||||

Insulin: The Two-Faced Hormone

The hormone insulin is like your pack-rat grandmother: It likes to store stuff. The only problem is that it's also as schizophrenic as old Uncle Judd. Sometimes it makes your muscles grow; sometimes it makes your fat cells grow.

Different foods create different insulin responses. Foods that have high–glycemic index rankings (including white bread, most cereals, grapes, and bananas) dump a lot of sugar into your bloodstream soon after you eat them, causing insulin levels to spike. In this case, insulin works quickly to turn that blood sugar into fat.

Some foods, though, cause a different reaction. Dairy products—milk, yogurt, ice cream—create dramatic insulin surges without the corresponding effect on blood sugar. You also get this insulin response from some foods that are virtually carbohydrate free, such as beef and fish, which have hardly any effect on blood sugar. When blood sugar remains relatively constant, it allows insulin to use the nutrients in your blood to build and repair cells, including muscle tissue.

That's why the Abs Diet centers around high-fiber, nutrient-dense foods that are also the ones thought to be most useful for weight control. Most are moderate to high protein, some are high in dairy calcium, and those that are carb-based emphasize fiber and other important nutrients.

It's hard to generalize about which carbs are high on the GI list and which are low because glycemic index is simply a measure of time—that is, how long it takes 50 grams of the food's carbohydrates to turn into blood sugar, regardless of serving size. It's a measure, for instance, of the carb-to-sugar conversion time for a whole apple or watermelon, but it doesn't tell you how much carb is in one serving of the food. Nobody eats a whole watermelon anyway.

That's why one latest advancement in food science is to look at a meal's glycemic load (GL). The GL considers both the GI of a food and the amount of carbs in one serving of that food. It helps you gauge the glycemic effect, or the projected elevation of blood glucose, that food will cause.

The higher a food's GL, the more it will cause your blood sugar to spike, and the less control you'll have over your energy levels and your appetite. But considering the GL is only one aspect of creating a balanced diet. "It's better to have a high-GL diet than one full of saturated fat," says Jennie Brand-Miller, PhD, professor of human nutrition at the University of Sydney and author of the International Table of Glycemic Index and Glycemic Load. "Aiming for the lowest GL possible is not a good move because that means you'll be eating too little carbohydrate and too much fat—probably saturated fat." Instead, to maintain your body's best glycemic response, center your meals around foods with GLs of 19 or less and shoot for a GL of less than 120 for the whole day.

Sound confusing? It doesn't need to be. The Abs Diet Powerfoods and the Abs Diet recipes all have low to moderate glycemic loads. All you have to do is follow the plan. And on those occasions when you are stuck and need to choose between two or more foods, refer to the chart on page 55.

Calcium: The Future of Fat Fighting

YOU'VE SEEN MORE than enough milk mustaches to know that calcium strengthens your bones, but did you know that calcium can also flatten your belly? Researchers at Harvard Medical School showed that those who ate three servings of dairy a day—which in conjunction with other foods provides about 1,200 milligrams of calcium (about the daily recommendation)—were 60 percent less likely to be overweight. In studies at the University of Tennessee,

(continued on page 56)

||||||||||||||||||||||||||||||||||||||||||||||||||||||||||||||||||||||||||||||||||||||||||||||||||||||||||

One Truly Corrupt Carb

Play word association with high-fructose corn syrup, and if you're like me, you say, "Froot Loops." But when nutritionists play the same game, they spit out another word: obesity. HFCS is a man-made sweetener that's cheaper and sweeter than sugar. Food manufacturers love it because it enhances their profits, so they add it into an unbelievable number of foods. Cereal. Ketchup. Soda. Pasta sauce. Cookies. Even some meal replacement bars, which are supposed to be good for you, list HFCS way up high on the ingredients list.

We're talking about a processed sweetener that didn't even exist in the food chain until the 1970s. And HFCS is really, really, really bad for you. That's because it's packed with calories, but your body doesn't recognize these calories. In fact, HFCS shuts off your body's natural appetite control switches, so you can eat and eat and eat far beyond what your body would normally be able to handle. You probably know people who can down a 2-liter bottle of Coke in a single sitting. Well, guess what? Before HFCS was invented, humans couldn't do that. Our natural appetite control switches would kick in, detect the sugar we were consuming, and say "¡No más!" But by shutting off the switches that control appetite, HFCS—a true junk food—is making America fat. By the late 1990s, Americans were consuming about 62 pounds per person every year. That's 228 additional calories per person per day.

The problem with HFCS is not the corn syrup; it's the fructose—a sugar that occurs naturally in fruit and honey. Corn syrup is primarily made of glucose, which can be burned as a source of immediate energy; stored in your liver or muscles for later use; or, as a last resort, turned to fat. But unlike glucose, fructose isn't metabolized by your body as an immediate source of energy; it's metabolized into fat. While the small amount of fructose you get naturally through fruit and honey won't make you fat, eating HFCS is sort of like setting up an IV that pumps fat directly to your gut. One of the worst offenders is soft drinks: Soda consumption has doubled from 25 to 50 gallons per person per year in the past few decades. So the amount of HFCS we're getting is unprecedented, and many researchers think there's a direct link between the huge amount of HFCS we're consuming and the huge numbers we're seeing on the scale.

Go back to what you know about carbohydrates. When you eat any carbohydrate—whether it contains glucose or starch—your body releases insulin to regulate your body weight. First, it tries to push the carbs into your muscle cells to be used as energy and facilitates carb storage in the liver for later use. Then it suppresses your appetite. Finally, it stimulates production of another protein, leptin, which is manufactured in your fat cells. In essence, leptin helps regulate how much fat you store and helps increase your metabolism to keep your weight in check. Like the nosy neighbor who tries to tell you how to raise your kids, fructose screws up a system that was working perfectly fine without it. Fructose doesn't stimulate insulin and therefore doesn't increase the production of leptin—and that's the most important argument against fructose and HFCS: Without insulin and leptin, your body has no shut-off mechanism. You can drink 4 liters of Coke or down half a gallon of frozen yogurt, and your body thinks you haven't eaten since the last time Bill Gates borrowed money from his dad.

Soft drinks are one of the main sources of HFCS, but researchers tried to determine whether soda itself or HFCS was the problem. The verdict: HFCS. In a study in the *American Journal of Clinical Nutrition,* researchers took two groups of overweight people and had one group drink regular soft drinks while the other group drank diet soda (which contains no HFCS) for 10 weeks. The regular soda group gained weight and increased their body fat, as well as saw an increase in their blood pressure. The diet soda group consumed fewer calories than they normally would, lost weight, reduced body fat, and lowered blood pressure.

Even if you aren't a soda drinker, HFCS can still sneak up on you. Here's where nutritional labels come in handy. If a label says "sugar" or "cane sugar," the product contains sucrose, which is a 50/50 blend of glucose and fructose. That doesn't seem to be much of a problem. If HFCS is listed first or second, look at the chart on the nutrition label to see how much sugar the food contains. If it's just a gram or two, don't sweat it. But if you see a food that has 8 or more grams of sugar and HFCS is prominent on the list of ingredients, do what you do when you get turned down for a date: Move along to something else. The body can deal with a little of anything, but when your HFCS numbers start looking like SAT scores, that's when you're headed for trouble. Consult the substitution chart for low-maintenance fixes.

FOODS HIGH IN HFCS OR FRUCTOSE	REPLACE WITH
Regular soft drinks	Unsweetened sparkling water or diet soda
Commercial candy (like jelly beans)	Chocolate candy (check the label; some chocolate bars have HFCS)
Pancake syrup	Real maple syrup
Frozen yogurt	Ice cream
Fruit-flavored yogurt	Organic yogurt
Highly sweetened cereals	Sugar-free or low-sugar cereals
Pasta sauce	Sugar-free pasta sauce
Energy bars	HFCS-free energy bars

researchers put women on diets that were 500 calories a day less than what they were used to eating. Yup, the women lost weight—about 1 pound of fat a week. But when researchers put another set of people on the same diet but added dairy to their meals, their fat loss doubled, to 2 pounds a week. Same calorie intake, double the fat loss.

Calcium seems to limit the amount of new fat your body can make, according to the University of Tennessee research team. In another study conducted at the same lab, people who added three servings of yogurt a day to their diets lost 61 percent more body fat and 81 percent more stomach fat over 12 weeks than those who didn't eat yogurt. A study in Hawaii found that teens with the highest calcium intakes were thinner and leaner than those getting less calcium.

Some researchers speculate that dairy calcium helps fight fat because it increases the thermic effect of eating—in other words, you burn more calories digesting calcium-rich foods than you would if you ate something with equal calories but no calcium. That's one reason why calcium supplements, though good for bone building and other bodily functions, don't have the same effect as dairy—fewer calories to digest, so fewer calories to burn. For best effect, shoot for about 1,200 milligrams of calcium per day.

The Abs Diet recommended calcium-rich foods are:

► 1 ounce grated Parmesan cheese (314 milligrams)

► 1 cup large-curd low-fat cottage cheese (126 milligrams)

► 8 ounces low-fat yogurt (415 milligrams)

► 8 ounces low-fat milk (264 milligrams)

► 1 ounce (1-inch cube) low-fat Swiss cheese (224 milligrams)

► 1 ounce (1 slice) low-fat Cheddar cheese (204 milligrams)

► 1 ounce low-fat mozzarella cheese (143 milligrams)

► 1 scoop (28 g) whey powder protein (110 milligrams)

Chapter 5

A FLAT BELLY IN 6 WEEKS

A Week-by-Week Guide to How Your
Body Will Change

I F YOU FLIP THROUGH THIS
book, you'll meet some of the people who went on the Abs Diet—and succeeded.
Linda Toomey lost 20 pounds while caring for four young kids. Rebecca Carr
became an athlete. And Jessica Guff stopped skipping meals—and started
wearing skimpier tops.

Everyone's body is different, and everybody who tries this plan will have a
different starting point. But based on the scientific research I've outlined, you
can lose up to 20 pounds of fat on the 6-week plan and gain up to 2 or 3 pounds
of muscle. For the average woman, that's enough of a transformation to have
your abs show. One of the bigger challenges, however, is monitoring your progress on the plan. Here's a look at the four major measurements you can use to
see just how effectively the Abs Diet will work for you.

Weight. It's the most straightforward. The heavier you are, the more at
risk you are for disease and the less fit you are. It's a good measuring stick to

(continued on page 62)

What the Heck Is . . . High Cholesterol?

Cholesterol is a soft, waxy substance found among the lipids (fats) in the bloodstream and in all your body's cells. For all the bad press it gets, the fact is that you need cholesterol because your body uses it to form cell membranes, create hormones, and perform several other crucial maintenance operations. But a high level of cholesterol in the blood—hypercholesterolemia—is a major risk factor for coronary heart disease, which leads to heart attack.

You get cholesterol in two ways. The body—mainly the liver—produces varying amounts, usually about 1,000 milligrams a day. But when you consume foods high in saturated fats—particularly trans fats—your body goes cholesterol crazy, pumping out more than you could ever use. Some foods also contain cholesterol, especially egg yolks, meat, poultry, fish, seafood, and whole-milk dairy products. But the majority of it, and the stuff I want you to focus on, is made by your own body.

Some of the excess cholesterol in your bloodstream is removed from the body through the liver. But some of it winds up exactly where you don't want it—along the walls of your arteries, where it combines with other substances to form plaque. Plaque is wack for several reasons: First, it raises blood pressure by making your heart work harder to get blood through your suddenly narrower vessels, which can eventually wear out your ticker. Second, plaque can break off its little perch and tumble through your bloodstream, eventually forming a clot that can lead to stroke, paralysis, death, and other annoyances.

Inside your body, a war is raging right now between two factions of specialized sherpas called lipoproteins that are moving cholesterol around your insides according to their own specialized agendas. There are several kinds, but the ones to focus on are the Jekyll and Hyde of health, HDL (high-density or "helpful" lipoprotein) and LDL (low-density or "lazy" lipoprotein) cholesterol.

The good guy: HDL cholesterol. About one-fourth to one-third of blood cholesterol is carried by helpful HDL. HDL wants to help you out by picking up cholesterol and getting it the hell out of your bloodstream by carrying it back to the liver, where it's passed from the body. That's good. Some experts believe that HDL removes excess cholesterol from plaques and thus slows their growth. That's really good. A high HDL level—above 60 milligrams per deciliter (mg/dL)—seems to protect against heart attack. The opposite is also true: A low HDL level—less than 40 milligrams per deciliter (mg/dL)—indicates a greater risk. A low HDL cholesterol level may also raise stroke risk.

The bad guy: LDL cholesterol. Lazy LDL has no interest at all in helping you out. LDL just wants to stick cholesterol in the most convenient place it can find, meaning your arteries. LDL doesn't care that too much cholesterol lining your arteries causes a buildup of plaque, a condition known as atherosclerosis. A high level of LDL cholesterol (160 mg/dL and above) reflects an increased risk of heart disease. Lower levels of LDL cholesterol reflect a lower risk of heart disease.

The other bad guy: triglycerides. These are a kind of fat in your blood that your body uses for energy. You need it, but when you have too much, you increase your risk for abdominal fat, diabetes, high blood pressure, even low HDL. A triglyceride check should be part of your regular cholesterol blood work. Ask for it if it isn't. A good triglyceride level is below 150 mg/dl. Triglycerides rise when you eat more calories than you burn off, drink a lot of alcohol or consume trans fats typically found in baked goods and chips.

Simply put, HDL is trying to come to your aid, while LDL and excess triglycerides are just sitting there, laughing at you. So whose side are you on? If you want to lower your triglycerides and boost HDL, start stocking up on the Abs Diet Powerfoods and follow the guidelines of the Abs Diet Workout. Here are some more quick ideas on beating the bad guys for good.

Drop 10 pounds. For every pound of fat you lose, your good HDL rises 1 percent.

Get him to butt out. You don't smoke; that's great! But if your partner does, your HDL could suffer. A recent study at Florida State University found that exposing nonsmokers to tobacco smoke in a typical tavern depressed their HDL levels up to 20 percent for up to two days.

Drink up or quit. In some studies, moderate use of alcohol is linked with higher HDL cholesterol levels. But take it easy there. People who consume moderate amounts of alcohol (an average of one drink per day for women) have a lower risk of heart disease, but increased consumption of alcohol can bring other health dangers, such as alcoholism, high blood pressure, obesity, and cancer. And alcohol raises triglyceride levels. If you have high tris, cutting out drinking alcohol is a sure way to bring them down.

Johnny B good. A B vitamin called niacin reduces LDL cholesterol at the same time it raises beneficial HDL. In fact, niacin can be more effective at treating these things than popular cholesterol-busting drugs, which tend to act more generally on total cholesterol and gross LDL. Be careful, though. While the niacin you get from foods and over-the-counter vitamins is fine, superhigh doses of niacin can have serious side effects and should be taken only under a doctor's supervision.

What the Heck Is . . . High Cholesterol? (cont.)

Tea it up. Three recent studies confirm that drinking green tea can help lower your cholesterol level and reduce your risk of developing cancer. In a 12-week trial of 240 people, researchers at Vanderbilt University found that drinking the equivalent of 7 cups of green tea a day can help lower LDL cholesterol levels by 16 percent. Seven cups a day is a lot of tea, but even 1 or 2 cups a day could have a beneficial impact. Meanwhile, researchers at the University of Rochester in New York recently determined that green tea extract can help prevent the growth of cancer cells, and Medical College of Ohio researchers found that a compound called EGCG in green tea may help slow or stop the progression of bladder cancer.

Go for the grapefruit. If you want to make one simple dietary change for better health, the best thing you can do is eat a single white or ruby grapefruit every day. New research shows that grapefruit can fight heart disease and cancer, trigger your body to lose weight, and even help you get a better night's sleep. A grapefruit a day can lower your total cholesterol and LDL levels by 8 and 11 percent, respectively.

Take a hike. Studies at Auburn University and the Cooper Institute in Dallas show that regular moderate exercise boosts HDL levels and reduces artery inflammation.

Cram in the cranberry. Researchers at the University of Scranton in Pennsylvania found that people who drank three glasses of cranberry juice daily raised their HDL cholesterol levels by 10 percent, which in turn lowered their risk of heart disease by 40 percent. Plant compounds called polyphenols are believed to be responsible for the effect. (Note: Cranberry juice often comes diluted, so make sure the label says that it contains at least 27 percent cranberry juice.)

Spread some on. Instead of butter or margarine, try Benecol spread. It contains stanol ester, a plant substance that inhibits cholesterol absorption. A study at the Mayo Clinic found that people eating 4½ tablespoons of Benecol daily lowered their LDL cholesterol by 14 percent in 8 weeks. When they stopped using it, their LDL returned to previous levels. Benecol can also be used for cooking.

Gain with grains and beans. Researchers at St. Michael's Hospital in Toronto had people add several servings of foods like whole grains, nuts, and beans to their diets each day. One month later, the test subjects' LDL cholesterol levels were nearly 30 percent lower than when the trial began. In another study, this one at Tulane University in New Orleans, researchers found that people who ate four or more servings a week had a 22 percent lower risk of developing heart disease (and 75 percent fewer camping companions) than less-than-once-a-week bean eaters.

Don't let your tank hit empty. A study in the *British Medical Journal* found that people who eat six or more small meals a day have 5 percent lower cholesterol levels than those who eat one or two large meals. That's enough to shrink your risk of heart disease by 10 to 20 percent.

Refrain from fries. In a study published in the *New England Journal of Medicine,* the exercise and nutritional habits of 80,000 women were recorded for 14 years. The researchers found that the most important correlate of heart disease was the women's dietary intake of foods containing trans fatty acids, mutated forms of fat that lower HDL and increase LDL. Among the worst offenders: french fries.

Sow oats. In a University of Connecticut study, people with high cholesterol who ate oat bran cookies daily for 8 weeks dropped their levels of LDL cholesterol more than 20 percent. So eat more oat bran fiber, such as oatmeal. The *American Journal of Clinical Nutrition* reports that two servings of whole-grain cereal (Cheerios count) a day can reduce your risk of dying of heart disease by nearly 20 percent.

Rise and dine. In a study of 3,900 people, Harvard researchers found that people who ate breakfast every day were 44 percent less likely to be overweight and 41 percent less likely to develop insulin resistance, both risk factors for heart disease.

Fortify with folate. A study published in the *British Medical Journal* found that people who consume the recommended amount of folate each day have a 16 percent lower risk of heart disease than those whose diets are lacking in this B vitamin. Good sources of folate include asparagus, broccoli, and fortified cereal.

Order a chef's salad. Leafy greens and egg yolks are both good sources of lutein, a phytochemical that carries heart disease–fighting antioxidants to your cells and tissues.

Be a sponge. Researchers at Loma Linda University in California found that drinking five or more 8-ounce glasses of water a day could help lower your risk of heart disease by up to 60 percent—exactly the same drop you get from stopping smoking, lowering your LDL cholesterol numbers, exercising, or losing a little weight.

Give yourself bad breath. In addition to lowering cholesterol and helping to fight off infection, eating garlic may help limit damage to your heart after a heart attack or heart surgery. Researchers in India found that animals that were fed garlic regularly had more heart-protecting antioxidants in their blood than animals that weren't.

Crank up the chromium. According to new research from Harvard, people with low levels of chromium in their systems are significantly more likely to develop heart problems. You need between 200 and 400 micrograms of chromium per day—more than you're likely to get from your regular diet. Look for a supplement labeled chromium picolinate; it's the most easily absorbed by the body.

Snack on nuts. Harvard researchers also found that people who replaced 127 calories of carbohydrates—that's about 14 Baked Lay's potato chips—with 1 ounce of nuts decreased their risk of heart disease by 30 percent.

gauge how well you're progressing on your diet, but it's incomplete in that it doesn't take into account the amount of muscle you're going to develop over the course of a plan. Muscle weighs about 20 percent more than fat, so even a dramatic fat loss may not translate into a dramatic drop in body weight.

Body mass index (BMI). The BMI is a formula that takes into consideration your height and your weight and gives you an indication of whether you're overweight, obese, or in good shape. To calculate your BMI, multiply your weight in pounds by 703, and divide the number by your height in inches squared. For example, let's say you are 5 feet 4 inches tall (that's 64 inches) and weigh 155 pounds. So first we multiply your weight by 703.

155 × 703 = 108,965

Next, we calculate your height in inches squared, meaning we multiply the number by itself.

64 × 64 = 4,096

Now we divide the first number by the second.

108,965 ÷ 4,096 = 26

That's not terrible. A BMI between 25 and 30 indicates you're overweight. Over 30 signifies obesity.

This measurement, too, has flaws. It doesn't take into account muscle mass, and it also leaves out another important factor—weight distribution; that is, where most of the fat on your body resides. But BMI can give you a pretty good idea of how serious your weight problem is.

Waist-to-hip ratio. Researchers have begun using waist size and its relationship to hip size as a more definitive way to determine your health risk. This is considered more important than BMI because of that visceral fat I talked about earlier—the fat that pushes your waist out in front of you. Because abdominal fat is the most dangerous fat, a lower waist-to-hip ratio means fewer health risks. To figure out your waist-to-hip ratio, measure your waist at your belly button and your hips at the widest point (around your butt). Divide your waist by your hips. For example, if your hips measure 36 inches and your waist at belly button level measures 30 inches, your waist-to-hip ratio is 0.83.

30 ÷ 36 = 0.83

That's not bad, but it's not ideal. Women want a waist-to-hip ratio of lower than 0.80. If you were to lose just 2 inches off your waist—something you can do in just 2 weeks with the Abs Diet—you'd find yourself in the fit range.

28 ÷ 36 = 0.77

Body fat percentage. Though this is the most difficult for the average person to measure because it requires a bit of technology, it's the most useful in terms of gauging how well your diet plan is working. That's because it takes into account not just weight but how much of your weight is fat. Many gyms offer body fat measurements through such methods as body fat scales or calipers that measure the folds of fat at several points on your body. See your local gym for what options they offer. Or try an at-home body fat calculator. I like the Taylor Body Fat Analyzer and Scale 5553 for its price (about $50), convenience, and accuracy. If you want a simple low-tech test (and this isn't as accurate as what the electronic versions will give you), try this simple exercise: Sit in a chair with your knees bent and your feet flat on the floor. Using your thumb and index finger, gently pinch the skin on top of your right thigh. Measure the thickness of the pinched skin with a ruler. If it's ¾ inch or less, you have about 14 percent body fat—quite fit for a woman. If it's 1 inch, you're probably closer to 18 percent fat, which is also very desirable for a woman. If you pinch more than an inch, you could be at increased risk for diabetes and heart disease.

Body fat percentage can be the most significant measurement because it'll really help give you a sense of how well you're sticking to a plan. As you see your body fat percentage decrease, you'll see an increase in the amount of visible muscle. Experts say that in order for your abs to show, your body fat needs to be about 12 percent. That means cutting body fat by a little more than half for the average woman.

Before you start the plan, it's important to record some of these measurements so that you'll know how far you're progressing. Take one baseline measurement, and then remeasure as needed for motivation. I'd recommend measuring every 2 weeks. That'll be enough time to see significant differences to propel you through the next 2 weeks. (Measure body fat percentage only at the beginning and end of the plan, unless you have easy access to a measurement system.) Any sooner than that, and you're focusing too much on numbers rather than process.

MEASUREMENT	START	WEEK 2	WEEK 4	WEEK 6
Weight	131.4 +29.8			
BMI	22.9			
Waist-to-hip ratio				
Body fat percentage*				

Make sure to have the same person administer body fat readings using the same method to ensure consistency.

As with any diet plan, it's also important to develop some kind of quantitative goal—your ideal weight, waist size, or percentage of body fat. The chart above will help you figure out where you need to go.

ABS DIET SUCCESS STORY

"Off Came the Inches"

Name: Brandee Bratton

Age: 31

Height: 5'1"

Starting weight: 113

6 weeks later: 106

For Brandee Bratton, it was the perfect team approach: She would plan the food and meals, and her husband planned the workouts. What started out as a diet actually became more of a hobby, as the two made the program something they could do together. Starting at 113 pounds, Bratton didn't need to lose a lot of weight, but she still wanted something out of the Abs Diet.

"It's one thing to be petite, another to be strong, fit, healthy, and petite," she says.

So Bratton and her husband jumped on the program (he lost 10 pounds in 6 weeks), and Bratton wound up as a top-10 finalist in the initial Abs Diet Challenge—based

What's Your Perfect Weight?

IF YOU'RE LIKE a lot of the women I know, you hold one pivotal number in your brain. Not the date of your anniversary or the time your child was born or the number of calories in Mom's meat loaf. It's your ideal weight, a magical number that your mind fixates on as the one that you're truly meant to see when you step on the scale. Maybe you came to that number because it was your weight at age 18, or maybe it was your weight just before you got pregnant, or maybe it's the weight you think you would be if you could just drop that last little extra flab. Whatever the inspiration, you keep thinking that if you could only reach that goal, all your body-image woes would be over forever.

Well, as I've just outlined, weight certainly isn't the perfect measurement system. A lot of things play a role in how healthy you are—from your waist size to your amount of muscle mass. And that means that the number of pounds you weigh can be more misleading than a funhouse mirror. That said, you can

---

largely on the way she transformed the shape of her body.

"For the first 2 weeks, I didn't notice much of a change in terms of weight. What started changing was the inches, and then the pounds just came off at the end—mostly in the thighs and hips area," says Bratton, who also dropped from about 18 percent body fat to 12. "And that was when I really got excited."

Bratton, who enjoyed the interval training and healthy eating, says that the Abs Diet is one that anyone can follow because you're always satisfied.

"This diet isn't a fad diet; it follows all the scientific rules in terms of what to eat and how to eat," she says. "I can say that there's no food depri-

vation you feel through this. By eating six times a day, you feel satisfied. When it's time to eat, your body gets used to eating at that time, and your body lets you know—almost like it's talking to you: 'Hey, it's been 2 hours; give me something to eat.'"

Now Bratton, who feels healthier, stronger, and likes the new toned look of her body, is studying to become a personal trainer.

"Women often look for solutions through pills, milk in a can, and gadgets," she says. "I advise this program for any woman to invest in her body."

come pretty close to estimating your true ideal weight—not necessarily the one blinking on your brain's internal scoreboard but one that takes into consideration a number of different physical factors, including your body type and bone structure. While there's no absolute formula for predicting an exact ideal weight for every woman, the following formula will get you pretty darn close.

Step 1: Do the math. To get a baseline target weight, take the number of inches you are over 5 feet tall, multiply that number by 5, and add the total to 100 for a rough initial estimate of what someone of your height should weigh. So if you're 5 feet 4 inches, multiply 4 by 5 and add 100. Your baseline is 120. But you still need to factor in the other elements that contribute to your perfect weight.

YOUR BASELINE WEIGHT: _____%

Your frame can run large or small, no matter how tall you are. Researchers now recognize that having a large frame can add up to 10 pounds of healthy, unavoidable weight to your body. Take that baseline figure you just arrived at and adjust accordingly—5 to 10 pounds more for a large frame, 5 to 10 pounds less for a small frame, no adjustment necessary for a medium frame (see the chart below).

HEIGHT	WRIST CIRCUMFERENCE	FRAME SIZE
Under 5'2"	Under 5½"	Small
	Under 6"	Medium
	Under 6¼"	Large
Between 5'2" and 5'5"	5½" to 5¾"	Small
	6" to 6¼"	Medium
	6¼" to 6½"	Large
Over 5'5"	Over 5¾"	Small
	Over 6¼"	Medium
	Over 6½"	Large

YOUR BASELINE WEIGHT ADJUSTED FOR BONE STRUCTURE: _____

A body fat percentage of between 20 and 31 percent is considered a "normal" range for women (though as discussed on page 63, you have to be under that to have your abs show). If you can't use calibration tools, but you want a more precise gauge than the thigh-pinch method described on page 63, you can get a good estimation of your fat and how much of it you need to lose by using this formula: First, multiply your BMI (as determined using the formula on page 62) by 1.20. For our sample 155-pound woman, that's:

1.20 × 26 = 31.2

Then, multiply your age by 0.23. So the equation for a 26-year-old woman would be:

0.23 × 26 = 5.98

Add those two numbers together.

31.2 + 5.98 = 37.18

Subtract 5.4 from that number to find your body fat percentage.

37.18 - 5.4 = 31.78

YOUR BODY FAT PERCENTAGE: _____%

Use the following chart to determine how far over the goal you are. At almost 32 percent body fat, our sample woman is carrying 39 percent more fat than the ideal of 21 percent.

BODY FAT PERCENTAGE	PERCENT OVER GOAL
22	4
23	7
24	11
25	14
26	18
27	21
28	25
29	29
30	32
31	36
32	39

BODY FAT PERCENTAGE	PERCENT OVER GOAL
33	43
34	46
35	50
36	54
37	57
38	61
39	64
40	68
41	71
42	75
43	79
44	82

Translate your body fat percentage into how much sheer fat you're carrying around by multiplying your body fat by your current weight.

155 × 32% = 49.6, MEANING 49.6 POUNDS OF OUR 155-POUND WOMAN COMES FROM FAT

YOUR WEIGHT FROM FAT _____

Finally, multiply your percentage over goal from the chart by your total body fat. That's how many pounds of fat you should seek to lose.

49 × 39% = 19.11 POUNDS

Researchers at the New York Obesity Research Center at St. Luke's–Roosevelt Hospital found that waist size correlates better than overall body mass to risk factors for heart disease, such as high blood pressure, blood sugar, and cholesterol. To calculate your waist size, wrap the tape measure around the top of your hip bones. Take the measurement at the end of a normal breath. Then place your index finger next to your belly button and, standing up straight, see how many inches of belly fat you can grasp between your index finger and thumb. If your waist is more than 33 inches and you can pinch 2 inches of fat, you need to lose at least 10 pounds from your current weight, no matter how you've scored in other tests. If you can pinch 1 inch, you need to lose at least 5 pounds.

YOUR BELLY FAT: _____

Your "perfect weight" is somewhere between your baseline weight as adjusted for bone structure and the amount of weight you need to lose as determined by your weight from total body fat and the amount of belly fat you pinched.

Step 2: Change your calories. To consume fewer calories than you burn, it helps to know your metabolic rate—the number of calories you burn throughout the day. Most women have a metabolic rate of just under 1 calorie per minute, or about 1,440 calories per day. To determine your individual metabolic rate and daily calorie needs, multiply your weight in pounds by 11 to get your basic calorie needs (how much your body burns just by existing). So for our sample woman, that would be:

155 × 11 = 1,705

Then multiply your basic calorie needs by 1.6 to estimate your resting metabolic rate (rate of calories burned when you factor in your daily activities).

1,705 × 1.6 = 2,728

Next, factor in your exercise by multiplying the number of minutes per week that you run, cycle, or play sports by 8. As for strength training, if you're doing two sets of the Abs Diet Circuit, add 600 to your previous exercise total. If you're doing three sets, add 840. Divide the result by 7. Then add that number to your resting metabolic rate to get your total daily calorie needs. Here's the math for our sample woman if she does no cardio but does do two sets of the Abs Circuit.

600 ÷ 7 = 85.71

2,728 + 85.71 = 2,813

To get your estimated daily calorie budget if you want to lose 2½ pounds per week, subtract 1,250 from your total daily calorie needs.

2,813 - 1,250 = 1,563

Start off reducing your daily calorie intake much lower than that, and

(continued on page 72)

What the Heck Is . . . Diabetes?

Diabetes is a devastating disease that is reaching epidemic proportions. Twenty-four million Americans are living with diabetes and 10.2 percent of all women ages 20 years or older have the disease. A 2009 study at the University of Chicago forecasts that the population of Americans living with diabetes—both diagnosed and undiagnosed—will rise to 44 million people by 2034. Diabetes is the seventh leading cause of death in the US, but because it often goes undiagnosed, it is probably responsible for many more deaths. It's a leading cause of heart disease, kidney disease, and stroke, and its other complications include blindness, amputation, sexual dysfunction, and nerve damage. According to the Centers for Disease Control, someone with diabetes is twice as likely to die as someone the same age without diabetes. Fortunately, type 2 diabetes is also highly preventable (even reversible) and the Abs Diet and the Abs Diet Workout are near-perfect prescriptions.

Diabetes works like this: Your digestive system turns brunch into glucose—the form of sugar your body uses for energy—and sends it into the bloodstream. When the glucose hits, your pancreas—a large gland located near your stomach—produces insulin, a hormone, and sends that into the bloodstream as well. Insulin is your body's air traffic controller: It takes command of all your glucose and directs it into your cells, where it can be used for rebuilding muscle, for keeping your heart pumping and your brain thinking, or for doing the macarena (if you're the type to do the macarena, that is).

But over time, bad health habits can take a toll on your flight command center. Overeating, particularly eating high–glycemic index foods, floods your body with massive amounts of glucose time and time again. Like any air traffic controller, insulin can become overwhelmed when it's asked to do too much all at one time, and eventually it burns out. Insulin loses its ability to tell cells how to properly utilize the glucose in your blood—a condition known as insulin resistance. After several years, the pancreas gets fed up with producing all that ineffective insulin and begins to produce less than you need. This is called type 2, or adult-onset, diabetes. (Type 1, formerly known as juvenile diabetes, is caused by a defect in the pancrease.) Given that poor diet is the major risk factor for type 2 diabetes, it's no surprise that 80 percent of people with the disease are overweight. Glucose builds up in the blood, overflows into the urine, and passes out of the body. Thus, the body loses its main source of fuel even though the blood contains large amounts of glucose.

Two bad things happen: First, you start to lose energy, and your body starts to have trouble maintaining itself. You feel fatigue and unusual thirst, and you begin losing weight for no apparent reason; you get sick more often, and injuries are slow to heal because your body is losing its ability to maintain itself. Second, the sugar that is hanging around in your blood begins to damage the tiny blood vessels and nerves throughout your body, particularly in your extremities and vital organs. Blindness, sexual dysfunction, numbness, and heart damage ensue.

But type 2 diabetes is a preventable disease. Exercising and losing weight can reduce your risk by 60 percent, according to studies by the CDC, and—what a coincidence—that's just what this book is intended to teach you to do. So adopt the principles of the Abs Diet and the Abs Diet Workout, and, while you're at it, consider these additional steps.

C the Light. Women with the highest levels of vitamin C in their blood were 62 percent less likely than those with the lowest to develop diabetes, according to a 12-year-long study reported in 2009 in *Archives of Internal Medicine.* The researchers believe that the vitamin may prevent free radicals from damaging cells in a way that interferes with glucose metabolism. Women with the highest levels of vitamin C ate an average of 6.5 servings of fruits and veggies per day, so stock up on C sources like papayas, strawberries, oranges, cantaloupe, red bell peppers, and broccoli.

Get mushy. Oatmeal is high in soluble fiber, which may decrease your risk of heart disease, some cancers, diverticulitis, and diabetes. Mix it up: Eat oatmeal with berries and nuts one day, and have eggs and meat another.

Climb. Yale researchers found that people with insulin resistance—a risk factor for diabetes and heart disease—who exercised on a stairclimber for 45 minutes 4 days a week improved their sensitivity to insulin by 43 percent in 6 weeks.

Cruise the Mediterranean. Eating a Mediterranean-style diet—that is, whole grains, fresh vegetables and oily fish—maximizes your metabolism and slashes diabetes risk. A 2008 study of 13,380 people published in the *British Medical Journal* showed that those who adhered closely to a Mediterranean diet had a 35 percent lower risk of diabetes than those who did not consistently follow such an eating style.

Eat the right carbs. Get to know the glycemic index, a measure of how quickly the carbohydrates in a particular food are converted to glucose and released into the bloodstream. In a Harvard study, people who ate foods with the lowest indexes, such as whole-wheat bread, were 37 percent less likely to develop diabetes than those who ate high–glycemic index foods such as white rice. (To find out the glycemic index of various foods, go to www.glycemicindex.com or go to page 374.)

you'll lose more muscle than fat. As you begin to lose weight, though, deduct another 10 calories for every pound you drop.

I don't mean to hit you with more numbers than Paris Hilton's black book. In fact, it might be easiest to simply focus on one number—six—so that the others will fall into place. When you start to see those six abdominal muscles, it'll mean that everything else has decreased—your weight, your BMI, your waist-to-hip ratio, and your body fat percentage. This 6-week plan will get you there. Here's what you can expect from going on the diet.

WEEKS	WHAT TO EXPECT
1-2	A significant weight loss as your body adjusts to a new approach to eating. Some may see losses of up to 12 pounds in the first 2 weeks (especially if you're walking or otherwise active each day), but 5 to 8 pounds will be average.
3-4	By integrating a modest amount of strength training into your routine, you'll start to feel your body change because your metabolism is working hard. You'll notice an additional drop in weight (most likely averaging another 5 to 8 pounds), but you'll also notice significant changes in your shape.
5-6	After 2 weeks of exercise, your body is primed to make a significant push to drop more fat while also gaining muscle mass. You'll notice that your upper body is more toned and that your waist and other fatty parts of your body are smaller. Depending on your starting point, this is where you'll begin to see abs and really notice even greater effects.

What you'll find so remarkable about this program is how simple it is to follow, how often you'll eat—each meal and each snack is an easy, muscle-building, fat-burning treat—and how unlike any other "diet" the Abs Diet is. Very simply, the Abs Diet is a plan that will ask you to:

▶ Eat three meals and three snacks each day, with each of your meals and snacks including several of the wide-ranging powerfoods discussed in Chapter 8.

▶ Keep an eye out for a handful of diet busters that you'll learn to easily spot and cut down on—not eliminate.

▶ Perform a simple 20-minute workout three times a week to turbocharge your fat loss and muscle toning.

The Abs Diet is so simple that we don't break it into phases, and we didn't design a complex "maintenance" program (just a few simple words of wisdom that you'll find on page 359). The weight loss is yours to keep for life, and so is the eating plan. You won't be waiting for your "diet" to end. You'll enjoy this program so much—and be so wowed by the results—that you'll effortlessly follow it for life.

Chapter 6

SHOCKER: HOW LOW-CARB DIETS MAKE YOU FAT

The Truth about the Trend That's Threatening
America's Health

THROUGHOUT THIS BOOK, I've hit you with scientific evidence, persuaded you with real-life testimonials, and referenced study after study to show how the Abs Diet works and why it makes sense for everyone who wants to manage their weight and live healthful, active, disease-free lives. But, just for a moment, I want to step away from all the hard science and take you on a bit of a fantasy adventure. Come this way—I promise you'll find it revealing.

First, I want you to imagine that you've taken a time machine back to the Middle Ages. You find yourself at the door of an alchemist's laboratory, where magic elixirs and potions fill the shelves and the echoes of mantras and spells fill the air. You've traveled long and hard, through terrifying dark woods and vast, arid deserts to seek out a Holy Grail of sorts: a concoction that legend says will make you lose weight, magically.

The sorcerer appears, and he holds up before you two vials. The first, he says, contains an elixir that will protect you from most of the diseases known to man. Its ingredients hold properties that will change your cholesterol profile and protect you from heart disease; help scour your body for toxins and protect you from the onslaught of cancer and the side effects of aging; energize your body and your brain, making your thinking clearer and helping to immunize you from Alzheimer's; and, over the course of your long life, control your weight and keep obesity and diabetes at bay.

The second vial will do none of that. It will, in all likelihood, raise your cholesterol profile and increase your risk for cancer, stroke, and heart disease, as well as other ailments. But if you take it, it may help you lose weight dramatically—though only for a short period of time. And there's one more drawback: If you choose the second vial, you can never sip from the first.

Which do you choose?

In the past 10 years, more than 60 million Americans chose vial number two.

Now, scrape the dust from the label on that vial and guess what it says? Low-carbohydrate diet.

The first vial, on the other hand, brims with all sorts of things: fruits and vegetables, whole-grain breads and cereals, beans and nuts—the sorts of things that nature intended us to eat but diet plans like Atkins do not. And over the long term, if Americans keep choosing vial number two, I think we're going to pay—heavily.

The Origins of a Sweet Tooth

To UNDERSTAND WHY carbohydrates are important, we have to take another fantasy trip, this time back to the dawn of man. On the savannahs of Africa, the high plains of Europe, the wetlands of Asia, and the woodlands and jungles of the Americas, primitive man learned how to feed himself from nature's banquet table. He learned how to fish and hunt and, later, how to domesticate animals and grow grain. But since man first stood upright, he has also had a craving for sweets.

As with all things, there's a reason why we crave sweets. The sweetest things on earth, back in those days before Cherry Garcia, were fruits: wild berries, pears, citrus fruits, and the like. Not coincidentally, fruits are also packed with nutrients: vitamins to fend off disease; minerals to assist with cell function; and fiber to regulate hunger, control blood pressure, and help ease digestion. Without our sweet tooth, we would have been happy to eat nothing but woolly mammoth and buffalo meat—the original Atkins program. But nature saw to it that we craved the foods that would make us healthy.

Fast-forward to today, when the sweetest things don't look anything like tangerines. Whereas our sweet tooth was once nature's way of protecting us from disease, now it's the food industry's way of tricking us into it. To satisfy our cravings, we turn to cookies and cakes and chocolates instead of apples and pears and blackberries. That's one of the main reasons Americans today are so fat. And it's one of the main reasons why, in the short term, low-carb diets work.

By limiting carbohydrate intake, diets like Atkins create by default weight loss. If you restrict yourself to just one class of foods—low-carb foods, in this instance—you're bound to lose weight. That's because the stuff you're used to munching on, from the doughnut you nosh in the car on the way to work to the Snickers bar you snag from the vending machine before your drive home, is now voided from your diet. You're eating less food, so you're taking in fewer calories, so you lose weight.

The other sneaky advantage of an Atkins diet is that it focuses on foods that are difficult to prepare and consume. It's easy to pop a bagel or a grapefruit into your briefcase or purse; shove some steak and eggs in there instead, and things get a little messy. So low-carb diets restrict calories in two ways: by limiting food options and by limiting the ease with which we can consume food.

But there are two major reasons why, over the long term, low-carb diets won't work: Mother Nature and the almighty dollar.

Low-Carb Dilemma #1:
Take That Out of Your Mouth!

SOMEONE WITH A sound understanding of nutrition and a sadistic streak could have a field day torturing low-carb enthusiasts. Here's an evil trick: Take two pieces of soft, fresh, whole-grain bread. Slather one side with 2 tablespoons of all-natural peanut butter. Now take ½ cup of blackberries, mash them lightly with a fork, and (this is where it gets really nasty) spread the mashed berries onto the other piece of bread. Put the two sides together, and you've created the world's healthiest PB&J sandwich: 5 grams of fiber (about as much as the average American gets in a single day), 25 percent of your daily intake of vitamin C, 13 grams of protein, and (sacre bleu!) a verboten 30 grams of carbohydrate. (Oh, by the way, it tastes incredible.)

Float this concoction in front of a low-carb enthusiast, and you might as well be serving broiled rat viscera. (Come to think of it, they'd probably prefer the rat viscera. No carbs.) The sandwich is achingly sweet, soft, and chewy—a delicious comfort food that, at the same time, is a cholesterol-busting nuclear missile. The fiber protects you from heart disease as well as from stroke and colon cancer. The vitamin C boosts your immune system. And the high-quality (meaning high in fiber) carbs give you long-burning energy and food for your brain. Yet phase one of the Atkins diet bans every single ingredient in this simple sandwich.

Every single one.

In fact, the Atkins diet focuses on something called net carbs that Atkins claims are the carbohydrates that actually impact blood sugar. A rough formula for figuring out net carbs is to subtract the number of fiber grams from the total number of carb grams (the reasoning being that fiber doesn't impact blood sugar, spike insulin, or contribute to fat storage). By that calculation, this sandwich has about 33 net carbs. Phase one of the Atkins diet limits you to 20 net carbs per day. Eat this one super-good-for-you food, and you'll have to fast for the next day and a half to keep your Atkins diet in effect.

Maybe it's just me, but I think this whole low-carb plan is simply crackers. (Oh, sorry—not allowed to eat those.)

See, carbs are not our enemies. As I explained earlier, we crave carbs because we need them to protect us against a host of ailments. The low-carb craze works temporarily not because it limits carbs but because it limits food intake. And if I came out with some crazy diet plan that said you could eat only foods that are high in fat or low in protein or bigger than a bread box or start with the letter P, believe me—you'd lose weight. For a little while, at least, until you couldn't look at pudding, parsnips, and poultry ever again.

You'd lose weight because, by restricting your food intake, I've restricted your calorie intake. And the fact is, when you take in fewer calories than you burn, you lose weight; when you take in more calories than you burn, you gain weight. That's true regardless of where those calories come from. The Abs Diet works both by cutting the number of calories you take in through a sensible-but-satiating eating plan and by increasing the number of calories you burn away by improving your metabolic function. Fewer calories coming in here, a few more burned off there, and presto—weight loss. No magic, no deprivation, and no pointing fingers at the evils of carbohydrates.

The confusion about carbs comes from the fact that, in today's society, we're surrounded by high-carbohydrate foods that have had all their positive attributes stripped from them. The refined flours and sugars and sugar substitutes that you find in everything from cookies to ice cream to mass-produced ketchup and peanut butter give us all the calories and none of the nutritional benefits of their original ancestors: whole grains and fruits. The lack of fiber in, say, a plain bagel causes the calories in the bagel to be digested quickly, flooding the bloodstreams with glucose, triggering spikes in the digestive hormone insulin—which then turns the blood sugar into fat cells and leaves you hungry once again.

But fruits, vegetables, and whole-grain bread products have a very different effect on the body: They're digested slowly, giving us long-burning energy. Insulin levels stay steady while fiber scours our bodies for cholesterol and other harmful substances, and the vitamins and minerals inherent in those foods help protect us from a host of ills.

The longer we try to go without carbs, the more our bodies crave them. Eventually, you have to fall off a carb-restricting diet: Your body is programmed to make you seek out carbs, just the way it's programmed to blink when something hurtles toward your eye. It's one of our natural defense mechanisms, and what Mother Nature wants, she will eventually get.

Then again, what corporate America wants, it too will get. Which presents us with part two of why the low-carb craze is a disaster waiting to happen.

Low-Carb Dilemma #2: Follow the Money

REMEMBER WHAT I said about why the low-carb diet appears to work? Because it cuts out a majority of foods that people love to eat and because it makes eating on the run difficult. Those two factors conspire to restrict calories, and fewer calories mean less weight.

Now, here's an easy question: How do food manufacturers make money? By selling you food. So what happens when 60 million Americans decide they're going to stop buying all the candy bars, loaves of bread, boxes of pasta, and

jars of sugary spreads that manufacturers have obligingly loaded with carbohydrates over the past half century?

Food manufacturers are going to have to come up with something else to
sell. Something they can tout as low-carb, to appeal to Atkins-oriented dieters, but something that's familiar, easy to find, and even easier to consume.
And so begins the next phase in the American obesity epidemic.

In 2004, the *New York Times* reported on the growing trend toward low-
carb marketing among restaurants and grocery stores. Retailers were being
counseled by their business advisors to open up "low-carb" aisles; restaurants
were vying for the coveted "Atkins approved" label to hang in their windows.
And in the past 6 years, nearly 1,000 new food products claiming to be low in
carbohydrates have hit the shelves. Today, you can snack on low-carb candy,
low-carb cake, and low-carb brownies, washing it all down with a couple of
bottles of low-carb beer.

To get a sneak preview of where all this is going, let's hop back into that
time travel machine. This time, we're not going to the storied Middle Ages
or the dawn of humanity . . . we're just going back about 17 years or so, to the
beginnings of the last diet craze that swept the nation: the low-fat craze.

It's the early 1990s. The low-carb craze hasn't yet begun to blossom. (For
better or worse, neither has Britney Spears.) But another mantra has begun
to take hold in American society: Eat less fat.

This directive comes not from a book-peddling diet doc but from the US
government, in the form of a revised food pyramid designed by the Food and
Drug Administration. Fat has been fingered as the root of all dietary evils:
Simply put, fatty foods translate into fatty people. Diet experts race to defend
this idea, which on the face of it seems pretty logical: Dietary fat is more easily
transformed into body fat, whereas carbohydrates are preferentially burned
off for energy. Hence, swap your fat calories for carb calories, and voilà, you've
entered the magical weight loss zone.

Quickly, food manufacturers move to capitalize on these exciting develop-
ments. As sales of fat-free milk rise, packages of reduced-fat, low-fat, and fat-
free cheeses, spreads, yogurts, ice creams, cakes, and cookies begin to fill the
supermarket shelves. Some taste okay. Some taste like sugar-crusted card-
board. But what the heck—no fat, no foul. Carbo-loading becomes a byword of
amateur athletes all across the country.

However, this whole low-fat theory comes with one big but. (Actually, it comes with millions of big butts, as the obesity rate has risen more than 15 percent in the past decade.) Like today's low-carb craze, the low-fat craze originally appears to work because it creates a restrictive eating program that eliminates certain foods and, hence, a certain number of calories. If you suddenly have to cut out countless steaks, baked goods, slabs of butter, nuts, dairy products, and desserts, presto—you lose weight.

But, as with carbohydrates, our bodies crave fat. Fatty foods (beef, fish, and dairy products, for instance) are usually high in muscle-building proteins and supply critical vitamins and minerals (the vitamin E in nuts and oils, the calcium in cheese and yogurt). So you can go on a low-fat diet for only so long before you wind up facedown in a pint of Chunky Monkey. That's the way Mother Nature planned it.

What she didn't plan for, however, was the craftiness of food marketers. Knowing that low-fat dieters are secretly pining for the old days when a nice slice of cake and a scoop of ice cream ended every celebratory meal, grocery manufacturers go into the laboratory and come out with hundreds of new low-fat foods. And that leads to what should go down in history as The Great SnackWells Debacle.

Nabisco conceived SnackWell's as the ultimate answer to the low-fat diet craze. SnackWell's, which you can still find on grocery shelves today, are fat-free and low-fat cookies that somehow carry nearly all the flavor of full-fat cookies. The secret is that Nabisco loads up the cookies with extra sugar (except in the sugar-free varieties), so you can indulge your sweet tooth without ever missing the fat. How this development plays out in the mind of the average consumer is simple to predict.

"All I have to do to lose weight is to cut out fat."

"Hey! These cookies have no fat. Let's buy two packages!"

"Honey, did you eat that second package of cookies for breakfast? I wanted it!"

The magic bullet doesn't work, in part because we need to eat fats and in part because we've been fooled into thinking that we can eat whatever we want, in whatever quantity we want, as long as we aren't eating fat. So we scarf down sugar calories by the spoonful, and we all get just a little bit fatter in the process.

Okay, hop out of the time machine—trip's over. It's a decade later and, instead of a low-fat craze, America is caught up in the throes of a low-carb craze. And the same scenario is playing out all over again. Every grocery store and corner deli is filled with products—particularly "meal replacement" bars—that are marketed with bywords like low-carb or carb smart.

Suddenly, it's not hard to eat low-carb anymore. Today—and increasingly more so tomorrow—we can fill our shopping carts with all the foods we cut out for the past couple of years. Food marketers are altering the makeups of their products, packing them with soy protein and fiber and sugar alcohols—all ingredients that lower the "net carb" impact of the food. Now, I'm all for more protein and fiber. Sugar alcohol, on the other hand, is nothing but empty calories that, in elevated quantities, cause gastric distress and flatulence.

What I am against is the notion that marketers are peddling—that we can eat whatever and whenever we want as long as we're not eating carbs. It is exactly the same trap we fell into more than 10 years ago: a restrictive diet that offers short-term success, turned into a food craze that guarantees even greater health risks and higher obesity rates.

And that's a time travel destination no one wants to arrive at.

ABS DIET HEALTH BULLETIN

What the Heck Are . . . Cancer Cells?

Cancer is the one scourge that can strike any of us at any time in life. It can hit in the places we think about and care about on a daily basis—the skin, the lungs, the brain—or in obscure places we don't even understand, like the pancreas, the kidneys, or the lymphatic system.

Simply put, cancer develops when cells in one part of the body begin to grow out of control. When we're children, our cells are constantly dividing, creating the new cells that help us grow. Once we reach adulthood, that cell growth stops, for the most part. Once we reach our genetically programmed height and weight, cells in most parts of the body divide only to replace worn-out or dying cells or to repair injuries.

But cancer cells act like kids—they keep growing, dividing, and multiplying, outliving our normal cells and interfering with the various functions of the body. Cancer is the second-leading cause of death in the US; heart disease is number one. The most common type of cancer among women is breast cancer, resulting in about a quarter million new cases every year. It's the second most fatal cancer among women, preceded by lung cancer.

We don't fully understand what causes cancer, but we do know some of the risk factors: Obesity, low-fiber diets, smoking, heavy alcohol use, overexposure to the sun, and exposure to radiation and other toxins are among the biggest dangers. Additionally, there's a strong link between heredity and cancer; if one or more close relatives has suffered a bout of the disease, you're at increased risk for cancer in general and for that specific form in particular.

I'd like to tell you that the Abs Diet is a magic bullet against cancer, but I can't; while dietary changes and exercise can dramatically decrease your risk for heart disease, stroke, and especially diabetes, cancer remains a bit more elusive. Still, by adopting the principles of the Abs Diet, you'll automatically decrease your risk for many forms of cancer because you'll decrease your weight and increase your fiber intake. In the meantime, you can also follow these additional tips to slash your risk even more.

Trim the fat. The more fat you eat, the greater your risk of developing a highly fatal form of cancer. In a study of more than 500,000 people reported in the *Journal of the National Cancer Institute,* those who ate the most fat (about 40 percent of their daily calories) were 23 percent more likely to develop pancreatic cancer than those who ate the least (about 20 percent of their cals). Limit fat to 20 to 35 percent of your calories—about 40 to 70 grams total in an 1,800-calorie diet.

Go for yolk. Research in 2009 suggests that egg yolk may be cancer-protective. The yellow stuff is rich in choline, which has been linked to lower rates of breast cancer. One yolk delivers 25 percent of your daily needs.

Hail a cabbage. Each 22-calorie cup of cabbage is loaded with sulforaphane, a chemical that increases your body's production of the enzymes that disarm cell-damaging, cancer-causing free radicals.

Be like Popeye. A 2009 report in the *International Journal of Cancer* shows that people who ate the most folate-rich leafy greens, such as spinach, had half as many skin cancer tumors as those who ate the least. It's thought that the folate in greens may help repair DNA.

Bite a blackberry. It contains anthocyanins, powerful antioxidants that have been shown to fight various forms of cancer, according to a new study in *Cancer Prevention Research.*

Try the cheese platter. A large-scale study of 120,000 women found that premenopausal women who consumed a lot of dairy products, especially low-fat and fat-free ones, ran a lower risk of breast cancer.

Serve the salmon. Or any other fish high in omega-3 fatty acids. Omega-3s can help mollify your cancer risk.

Eat the whole grain. Whole-grain carbohydrates are a great source of fiber. European researchers found that those with the highest daily intakes of fiber also had a 40 percent lower risk of developing colon cancer.

Sip hot tea. A 2007 study in *The Journal of Nutritional Biochemistry* found that drinking 2 to 6 cups of hot green tea a day helps prevent skin cancer and may reverse the aging affects of the sun's rays. Drink it hot to reap the greatest amount of catechins, a type of antioxidant with proven anti-cancer properties.

Get a D. Foods high in vitamin D, like low-fat milk, help detoxify cancer-causing chemicals released during the digestion of high-fat foods, according to a study at the University of Texas Southwestern Medical Center.

Order drinks with a twist. According to University of Arizona research, lemon zest and orange zest contain d-limonene, an antioxidant that can reduce your risk of skin cancer by up to 30 percent if you consume quantities as small as 1 tablespoon per week.

Color your plate. A 14-year study found that those whose diets were highest in fruits and vegetables had a 70 percent lower risk of digestive-tract cancers.

Chapter 7

THE ABS DIET NUTRITION PLAN

The Powerfoods and System That Will Change Your Body

E ARLIER IN THE BOOK, I shared some cool science—how your body reacts to different foods, why some fats are good and others are evil, and how foods such as dairy products have a secret ingredient that helps your body burn fat. Science can be fun, but by this point in the book, you've probably got one burning question in your mind:

Hey, when can we eat?

So let's get right to it, because eating more of the right foods more often is the basis of the Abs Diet. Remember:

MORE FOOD + MORE MUSCLE = LESS FLAB

That's why the Abs Diet isn't a diet you'll feel you "have to" stick to. It's one you'll want to stick to.

Guideline 1: Eat Six Meals a Day

WE'RE SO USED to hearing people talk about eating less food that it's become weight-loss doctrine. But as you remember from the physiology of metabolism, you have to eat more often in order to change your body composition. The new philosophy that I want you to keep top of mind is "energy balance."

Researchers at Georgia State University developed a technique to measure hourly energy balance—that is, how many calories you're burning versus how many calories you're taking in. The researchers found that if you keep your hourly surplus or deficit within 300 to 500 calories at all times, you will best be able to change your body composition by losing fat and adding lean muscle mass. Those subjects with the largest energy imbalances (those who were over 500 calories in either ingestion or expenditure) were the fattest, while those with the most balanced energy levels were the leanest. So if you eat only your three squares a day, you're creating terrific imbalances in your energy levels. Between meals, you're burning many more calories than you're taking in. At mealtimes, you're taking in many more than you're burning. Research shows that this kind of eating plan is great—if your dream is to be a high-rise condo. But if you want to look slimmer, feel fitter, and—not coincidentally—live longer, then you need to eat more often. In the same study, subjects who added three snacks a day to three regular meals balanced out their energy better, lost fat, and increased lean body mass (as well as increased their power and endurance).

In a similar study, researchers in Japan found that athletes who ate the same amount of calories a day from either two or six meals both lost an average of 11 pounds in 2 weeks. But the ones who ate six meals a day lost 3 pounds more fat and 3 pounds less muscle than the ones who ate only two meals.

There's science to support the fact that more meals work, but the plain-speak reason it works is because it does something that many diets don't do: It keeps you full and satiated, which will reduce the likelihood of a diet-destroying binge.

How it works: For scheduling purposes, alternate your larger meals with smaller snacks. Eat two of your snacks roughly 2 hours before lunch and dinner, and one snack roughly 2 hours after dinner.

Sample time schedule:

> **8 a.m.: breakfast**
>
> **11 a.m.: snack**
>
> **1 p.m.: lunch**
>
> **4 p.m.: snack**
>
> **6 p.m.: dinner**
>
> **8 p.m.: snack**

For examples of weekly meal plans, check out Chapter 10. These plans are not something you need to stick to religiously, just a suggestion for how you can make the Abs Diet work for you. It also shows how to incorporate the recipes you'll find in Chapter 9 into your everyday life.

Guideline 2: Make These 12 Abs Diet Powerfoods the Staples of Your Diet

THE ABS DIET will teach you to focus on (not restrict yourself to) a handful of food types—the Abs Diet Power 12—to fulfill your core nutritional needs. These foods are all good for you. They're so good, in fact, that they'll just about single-handedly exchange your fat for a toned, lean body (provided you've kept your receipt). Just as important, I've designed the Power 12 to include literally thousands of food combinations. There are hundreds of dairy products, fruits and vegetables, lean meats, and other choices to satisfy your tastes. Incorporating these powerfoods into your six meals a day will satiate your tastes and cravings and keep you from feasting on the dangerous fat promoters in your diet.

You'll read more about these powerfoods in Chapter 8. For now, I just want you to remember:

A lmonds and other nuts

B eans and legumes

S pinach and other green vegetables

D airy (fat-free or low-fat milk, yogurt, cheese)

I nstant oatmeal (unsweetened, unflavored)

E ggs

T urkey and other lean meats

P eanut butter

O live oil

W hole-grain breads and cereals

E xtra-protein (whey) powder

R aspberries and other berries

Guideline 3: Drink Smoothies Regularly

WITH SCHEDULES THE way they are today, it's no wonder that your definition of a kitchen appliance is the take-out menu. No matter how busy you are, you need to squeeze one appliance into your life: the blender. I don't care how many speeds it has or how it looks, and I couldn't tell you the difference between a mince and a frappe. All I care about is how much stuff I can put in it and how good the stuff tastes when it comes out. (One thing I do recommend: Get a blender with at least 400 watts, which will give it the power to handle chopping ice and shredding fruit and to outlast any Jimmy Buffett fans who might drop by unexpectedly.)

When you consider that changing your body takes time, motivation, and knowledge, consider your blender to be one of your most powerful tools in this plan. Smoothies made with a mixture of the Abs Diet Powerfoods can act as meal substitutions and as potent snacks, and they work for a few reasons.

▶ They require little time.

▶ Adding berries, flavored whey powder, or peanut butter will make them taste like dessert, which will satisfy your sweet cravings.

▶ Their thickness takes up a lot of space in your stomach.

Here's the evidence showing these blended power drinks will help you control your weight.

▶ Researchers at Purdue University in West Lafayette, Indiana, found that people stayed fuller longer when they drank thick drinks than when they drank thin ones—even when calories, temperatures, and amounts were equal.

▶ A Penn State study found that people who drank yogurt shakes that had been blended until they doubled in volume ate 96 fewer calories a day than those who drank shakes of normal thickness.

▶ In a study presented at the North American Association of the Study of Obesity, researchers found that regularly drinking meal replacements increased the chances of losing weight and keeping it off for longer than a year.

▶ A University of Tennessee study found that people who added three servings of yogurt a day to their diets lost 61 percent more body fat and 81 percent more stomach fat over 12 weeks than those who didn't eat yogurt. Wow! Researchers speculated that the calcium helps the body burn fat and limit the amount of new fat your body can make.

How it works: Drink an 8-ounce smoothie for breakfast, as a meal substitute, or as a snack before or after your workout.

Guideline 4: Stop Counting

BY EATING THE 12 Abs Diet Powerfoods and their many relatives, the foods themselves will, in a way, count your calories for you. They'll keep you healthy and feeling full and satisfied. Plus, the most energy-efficient foods are almost like doormen at a nightclub: They're not going to let any of the riffraff in without your approval.

Of course, that doesn't give you license to speed down the road of monstrous portions. Most of us claim that we watch what we eat, but most of us don't have a clue. A US Department of Agriculture study asked people what they ate, then checked it against reality. The truth: People eat twice the grains, fats, and sweets that they estimate. If you eat six well-balanced meals, your body will regulate portions through things like fiber, protein, and the sheer volume of the smoothies. That said, it's always wise—especially in the beginning of the plan, when you're most vulnerable and adjusting to a new way of eating—to focus on portion control by limiting the servings of some foods, especially the ones with fat (like peanut butter) and carbohydrates (like rice or bread). A good rule: Stick to one to two servings per food group and keep the total contents of each meal contained to the diameter of your plate. A height restriction is in effect. If you do like to count calories, go at it. I'll give you some strategies for doing so on page 156.

Guideline 5: Know What to Drink— And What Not To

I DRINK BEER. I drink wine. I like to drink beer and wine, and gin and tonics on a hot summer day, and a lot of other things. There are health benefits to having one or two drinks a day, but there are many ways that alcohol can get you into trouble. Most important, alcohol—just like soda—adds calories that you don't need right now. These calories are empty calories because they don't actually help make you full or decrease the amount of food you'll eat. In fact, alcohol makes you eat more and encourages your body to burn less fat. When Swiss researchers gave eight healthy people enough alcohol to exceed their daily calorie requirements by 25 percent (five beers for someone who eats 3,000 calories a day), they found that booze actually impaired their ability to burn fat by as much as 36 percent. Booze also makes you store fat. Your body sees alcohol as a poison and tries to get rid of it. So your liver stops processing all other calories until it has dealt with the alcohol. Anything else you eat while you're drinking most likely will end up as fat. In some more indirect ways, alcohol can inhibit your body's production of hormones that help burn fat and build muscle.

I hate to tell you to drink water, but drinking about eight glasses a day has a lot of benefits. It helps keep you satiated. (A lot of times what we interpret as hunger is really thirst.) Water flushes the waste products your body makes when it breaks down fat for energy or when it processes protein. You also need water to transport nutrients to your muscles, help digest food, and keep your metabolism clicking.

If you're serious about shedding belly flab, I'd encourage you to stay away from alcohol for the 6-week plan. At the least, limit yourself to two or three alcoholic drinks per week. The best drinks you can have are fat-free, 1 percent, or 2 percent milk; water; and green tea (or, if you must, two glasses of diet soda a day).

Guideline 6: For One Meal a Week, Forget the First Five Guidelines

I WOULD NEVER advocate cheating on your spouse, your employer, or your taxes. But I want you to cheat on this diet. I want you to take one meal during the week and forget everything about good carbohydrates and good fats. Have half a pizza, Kit Kats, Alfredo sauce, or whatever it is that you miss the most while you're on this plan. Have it, savor it, and then dig back in for another week. I want you to cheat for a couple reasons. One, I want you to control when you cheat. Plan your cheat meal for the week—whether it's Saturday night out, a neighbor's cookout, or whenever. But if you keep it planned, you'll stick to it. The way to control your cravings is to satisfy them every once in a while. If you can make it through 6 days, you reward yourself and know that 6 days of good eating is a regimen you can stick to over the long term. And there's another important reason I want you to cheat: because it'll actually help you change your body. A successful diet plan is about how you eat most of the time, not how you eat all of the time. In fact, a high-calorie day of eating can rev up your metabolism. Researchers at the National Institutes of Health found that people who ate twice as many calories in a day as they normally did increased their metabolism by 9 percent in the 24-hour period that followed. But here's where you have to show control. I think that this diet plan allows you to have plenty of foods that are both good and good for you, but I know you will crave other foods that don't fit into our guidelines. Think of this cheat meal as the carrot at the end of a good week of eating. I encourage you to enjoy your meal of gluttony, and please, don't make the carrot literally a carrot.

‖‖

Extra Credit

Turbocharge the six Abs Diet guidelines by establishing these three simple habits of lean and healthy eating.

1. Prepare your own meals. As your number of home-cooked meals increases, your fast-food visits decrease. By cooking at home using the recipes in the next chapter, you'll automatically avoid huge restaurant portions and calorie overload. USDA scientists found that people eat about 500 calories more a day when they consume food made outside the home.

2. Eliminate added sugars. "This is the simplest way to clean up any diet," says Jonny Bowden, PhD, the author of *The 150 Healthiest Foods on Earth*. Avoid putting sugar in anything you eat. And stay away from soda, baked goods, fruit drinks, and sugary breakfast cereals. USDA researchers say 82 percent of our added sugar can be attributed to those foods.

3. Don't fear fat. Fats found in meat, dairy, avocados, olive oil, and nuts are filling and add flavor to meals, which will help you avoid feeling deprived, says nutritionist Alan Aragon, MS. For a rule of thumb, shoot for half a gram of fat for every pound of your desired body weight.

Chapter 8

THE ABS DIET POWER 12

Meet the Powerfoods That Will Shrink Your Belly
And Keep You Healthy for Life

I
N THE PREVIOUS CHAPTER,
I gave you the six guidelines for following the Abs Diet and touched briefly on the
Abs Diet Power 12. Now I want you to meet each of these 12 superheroes up close.

These 12 foods make up a large part of your diet. The more of these foods
you eat, the better your body will be able to increase lean muscle mass and
avoid storing fat. Though you can base entire meals and snacks around these
foods, you don't have to. But do follow these guidelines.

▶ Incorporate two or three of these foods into each of your three major
meals and at least one of them into each of your three snacks.

▶ Diversify your food at every meal to get a combination of protein,
carbohydrates, and fat.

▶ Make sure you sneak a little bit of protein into each snack.

How to read the key: For at-a-glance scanning, I've included the following icons under the descriptions of each of the Abs Diet Powerfoods. Each icon
demonstrates which important roles each food can help play in maintaining
optimum health.

Builds muscle: Foods rich in muscle-building plant and animal pro-teins qualify for this seal of approval, as do foods rich in certain miner-als linked to proper muscle maintenance, such as magnesium.

 Helps promote weight loss: Foods high in calcium and fiber (both of which protect against obesity) as well as foods that help build fat-bust-ing muscle tissue earn this badge of respect.

 Strengthens bone: Calcium and vitamin D are the most important bone builders, and they protect the body against osteoporosis. But beware: High levels of sodium can leach calcium out of bone tissue. Fortu-nately, all of the powerfoods are naturally low in sodium.

 Lowers blood pressure: Any food that's not high in sodium can help lower blood pressure—and score this designation—if it has beneficial amounts of potassium, magnesium, or calcium.

 Fights cancer: Research has shown that there is a lower risk of some types of cancer among those people who maintain low-fat, high-fiber diets. You can also help foil cancer by eating foods that are high in calcium,

||||||||||||||||||||||||||||||||||||||||||||||||||||||||||||||||||||||||||||||||||||||||||||||||||||

Obesity Risks

Almost as important as what you eat is when you eat. Researchers at the University of Massachusetts analyzed the eating habits of 500 women and men and found connections between the way people eat and the risk of becoming overweight.

HABIT	CHANGES YOUR RISK OF OBESITY BY
Eating at least one midday snack	–39 percent
Eating dinner as your biggest meal of the day	+6 percent
Waiting more than 3 hours after waking up to eat breakfast	+43 percent
Eating more than a third of your meals in restaurants	+69 percent
Going to bed hungry (3 or more hours after your last meal or snack)	+101 percent
Eating breakfast away from home	+137 percent
Not eating breakfast	+450 percent

beta-carotene, or vitamin C. In addition, all cruciferous (cabbage type) and allium (onion type) vegetables get the cancer protection symbol because research has shown they help prevent certain kinds of cancer.

 Improves immune function: Vitamins A, E, B6, and C; folate; and the mineral zinc help to increase the body's immunity to certain types of disease. This icon indicates a powerfood with high levels of one or more of these nutrients.

 Fights heart disease: Artery-clogging cholesterol can lead to trouble if you eat foods that are predominantly saturated and trans fats, while foods that are high in monounsaturated or polyunsaturated fats will actually help protect your heart by keeping your cholesterol levels in check.

#1: Almonds and Other Nuts

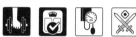

Superpowers: build muscle, fight cravings

Secret weapons: protein, monounsaturated fats, vitamin E, fiber, magnesium, folate (peanuts), phosphorus

Fight against: obesity, heart disease, muscle loss, wrinkles, cancer, high blood pressure

Sidekicks: pumpkin seeds, sunflower seeds, avocados

Imposters: salted or smoked nuts

These days, you hear about good fats and bad fats the way you hear about good cops and bad cops. One's on your side, and one's gonna beat you silly. Oreos fall into the latter category, but nuts are clearly out to help you. They contain the monounsaturated fats that clear your arteries and help you feel full.

All nuts are high in protein and monounsaturated fat. But almonds are like Jack Nicholson in *One Flew over the Cuckoo's Nest:* They're the king of the nuts. A handful of almonds provides half the amount of vitamin E you need in a day and 8 percent of the calcium. They also contain 19 percent of your daily requirement of magnesium—a key component for muscle building. In a Western Washington University study, people taking extra magnesium were able to lift 20 percent more weight and build more muscle than those who weren't.

Eat as much as two handfuls of almonds a day. A Toronto University study found that people can eat this amount daily without gaining any extra weight. A Purdue University study showed that people who ate nuts high in monounsaturated fat felt full an hour and a half longer than those who ate fat-free food (rice cakes, in this instance). If you eat 2 ounces of almonds (about 24 of them), it should be enough to suppress your appetite—especially if you wash them down with 8 ounces of water. The fluid helps expand the fiber in the nuts to help you feel fuller. Also, try to keep the nuts' nutrient-rich skins on them.

Here are ways to seamlessly introduce almonds or other nuts into your diet.

▶ Add chopped nuts to plain peanut butter.

▶ Toss a handful on cereal, yogurt, or ice cream.

▶ Put slivers in an omelet.

▶ For a quick popcorn alternative: Spray a handful of almonds with nonstick cooking spray and bake at 400°F for 5 to 10 minutes. Take them out of the oven and sprinkle with a mixture of either brown sugar and cinnamon or ground red pepper and thyme.

‖‖

Eat Beans, Stay Lean

Beans, beans, so good for your heart...but new research shows they're also good for your waistline and other body parts. People who eat ³⁄₄ cup of beans daily weigh 6.6 pounds less than those who don't eat beans, even though the bean eaters consumed 199 calories more a day, according to a presentation at a recent Experimental Biology Conference. Check out this bean dream team and what it can do for you.

The antiaging agent: red kidney beans. This chili staple contains more antioxidants and omega-3s than any of its bean brethren. Kidneys are also rich in thiamine, which research shows may be protective against Alzheimer's disease.

The heart healer: navy beans. These beans pack the most fiber of any at 10.5 grams per 100-gram serving, so they are powerful weapons against cholesterol. Also, kidneys are loaded with potassium, which regulates blood pressure and normal heart contractions. Almost neutral in taste, these beans absorb flavors well, so they are especially good for adding fiber and protein to soups and stews.

One caveat, before you get all nutty: Smoked and salted nuts don't make the cut here because of their high sodium content. High sodium can mean high blood pressure.

#2: Beans and Legumes

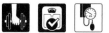

Superpowers: build muscle, help burn fat, regulate digestion

Secret weapons: fiber, protein, iron, folate

Fight against: obesity, colon cancer, heart disease, high blood pressure

Sidekicks: lentils, peas, bean dips, hummus, edamame

Imposters: refried beans, which are high in saturated fats; baked beans, which are high in sugar

Most of us can trace our resistance to beans to some unfortunately timed intestinal upheaval (third-grade math class, a first date gone awry). But beans are, as the song says, good for your heart; the more you eat them, the more

||||||||||||||||||||||||||||||||||||||||||||||||||||||||||||||||||||||||||||||||||||||||||||||||||||||||

The brain booster: black beans. No beans boost brainpower like black beans. That's because they are full of anthocyanins, compounds that have been shown to improve brain function. Toss them into breakfast burritos or cheese quesadillas.

The muscle builder: soybeans. Technically a legume, soybeans are one of the only common plant foods that contain complete protein, making them terrific muscle-building meat substitutes for vegetarians.

The cancer killer: lentils. Women who frequently eat lentils have a significantly lower risk of developing breast cancer, according to a study in the *International Journal of Cancer*. The Nurses' Health Study II, which monitors the lifestyles of 90,000 women, found that women who ate beans or lentils two or more times per week had a 34 percent lower risk of breast cancer than women who ate them less often.

The diabetes destroyer: garbanzo beans. Also known as chickpeas, garbanzos are high in fiber, which helps stabilize blood sugar, lowering the risk of type 2 diabetes. Add them to salads and soups. Chickpeas (mashed) are the main ingredient in hummus, a garlicky bean spread that's terrific on crackers or as a healthier substitute for mayonnaise on sandwiches.

you'll be able to control your hunger. Black, lima, pinto, garbanzo—you pick the bean (as long as it's not refried—refried beans are loaded with fat). Beans are a low-calorie food packed with protein, fiber, and iron—ingredients crucial for building muscle and losing weight. Gastrointestinal disadvantages notwithstanding, they serve as one of the key members of the Abs Diet cabinet because of all their nutritional power. In fact, you can swap in a bean-heavy dish for a meat-heavy dish a couple of times per week; you'll be lopping a lot of saturated fat out of your diet and replacing it with higher amounts of fiber.

#3: Spinach and Other Green Vegetables

Superpowers: neutralize free radicals, which are molecules that accelerate the aging process

Secret weapons: vitamins including A, C, and K; folate; minerals including calcium and magnesium; fiber; beta-carotene

Fight against: cancer, heart disease, stroke, obesity, osteoporosis

Sidekicks: cruciferous vegetables such as broccoli and brussels sprouts; green, yellow, red, and orange vegetables like asparagus, peppers, and yellow beans

Imposters: none, as long as you don't fry them or smother them in fatty cheeses

You know vegetables are packed with important nutrients, but they're also a critical part of your body-changing diet. I like spinach in particular because one serving supplies nearly a full day's worth of vitamin A and half of your vitamin C. It's also loaded with folate—a vitamin that protects against heart disease, stroke, and colon cancer. To incorporate it, you can take the fresh stuff and use it as lettuce on a sandwich or try stir-frying it with a little fresh garlic and olive oil.

Another potent power vegetable is broccoli. It's high in fiber and more densely packed with vitamins and minerals than almost any other food. For instance, it contains nearly 90 percent of the vitamin C of fresh orange juice and almost half as much calcium as milk. It is also a powerful defender against diseases such as cancer because it increases the enzymes that help detoxify carcinogens. Tip: With broccoli, you can skip the stalks. The florets have three times as much beta-carotene as the stems, and they're also a great source of other antioxidants.

If you hate vegetables, you can learn to hide them but still reap the benefits. Try pureeing them and adding them to marinara sauce or chili. The more you chop and puree vegetables, the more invisible they become and the easier it is for your body to absorb them. With broccoli, sauté it in garlic and olive oil, then douse it with hot sauce.

#4: Dairy (Fat-Free or Low-Fat Milk, Yogurt, Cheese, and Cottage Cheese)

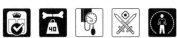

Superpowers: builds strong bones, fires up weight loss

Secret weapons: calcium, vitamins A and B12, riboflavin, phosphorus, potassium

Fights against: osteoporosis, obesity, high blood pressure, cancer

Sidekicks: none

Imposters: whole milk, frozen yogurt

Dairy is nutrition's version of a typecast actor. It gets so much attention for one thing it does well—strengthening bones—that it gets little or no attention for all the other stuff it does well. It's about time for dairy to accept a breakout role as a vehicle for weight loss. Just take a look at the mounting evidence: A University of Tennessee study found that dieters who consumed between 1,200 and 1,300 milligrams of calcium a day lost nearly twice as much weight as dieters getting less calcium. In a Purdue University study of 54 people, those who took in 1,000 milligrams of calcium a day (about 3 cups of fat-free milk) gained less weight over 2 years than those with low-calcium diets. Researchers think that calcium probably prevents weight gain by increasing the breakdown of body fat and hampering its formation. Low-fat yogurt, cheeses, and other dairy products can play an important role in your diet. But as your major source of calcium, I recommend milk for one primary reason: volume. Liquids can take up valuable room in your stomach and send the signal to your brain that you're full. Adding in a sprinkle of chocolate protein powder can also help curb sweet cravings.

#5: Instant Oatmeal
(Unsweetened, Unflavored)

Superpowers: boosts energy and sex drive, reduces cholesterol, maintains blood sugar levels

Secret weapons: complex carbohydrates and fiber

Fights against: heart disease, diabetes, colon cancer, obesity

Sidekicks: high-fiber cereals such as All-Bran and Fiber One

Imposters: cereals with added sugar and high-fructose corn syrup

Oatmeal is like a gold-medal routine on the balance beam—a perfect 10. You can eat it at breakfast to propel you through sluggish mornings, a couple of hours before a workout to feel fully energized by the time you hit the weights, or at night to avoid a late-night binge. I recommend instant oatmeal for its convenience. But I want you to buy the unsweetened, unflavored variety and use other powerfoods such as milk and berries to enhance the taste. Preflavored oatmeal often comes loaded with sugar calories.

Oatmeal contains soluble fiber, meaning that it attracts fluid and stays in your stomach longer than insoluble fiber (like vegetables). Soluble fiber is thought to reduce blood cholesterol by binding with digestive acids made from cholesterol and sending them out of your body. When this happens, your liver has to pull cholesterol from your blood to make more digestive acids, and your bad cholesterol levels drop.

Trust me: You need more fiber, both soluble and insoluble. Doctors recommend we get between 25 and 35 grams of fiber per day, but most of us get half that. Fiber is like a bouncer for your body, kicking out troublemakers and showing them the door. It protects you from heart disease. It protects you from colon cancer by sweeping carcinogens out of the intestines quickly.

A Penn State study also showed that oatmeal sustains blood sugar levels longer than many other foods, which keeps insulin levels stable and ensures you won't be ravenous for the few hours that follow. That's good, because spikes in the production of insulin slow metabolism and send a signal to the body that it's time to start storing fat. Because oatmeal breaks down slowly in the stomach, it causes less of a spike in insulin levels than foods like bagels. Include it in a smoothie or as your breakfast.

Another cool fact about oatmeal: Preliminary studies indicate that oatmeal raises the levels of free testosterone in your body, enhancing your body's ability to build muscle and burn fat, and boosting your sex drive.

#6: Eggs

Superpowers: build muscle, burn fat

Secret weapons: protein, vitamin B12, vitamin A

Fight against: obesity

Sidekicks: none

Imposters: none

Eggs contain the highest "biological value" of protein—a measure of how well it supports your body's protein need—of any food. In other words, the protein in eggs is more effective at building muscle than protein from other sources, even milk and beef. Eggs also contain vitamin B12, which is necessary for fat breakdown. Recent research from Louisiana State University showed that the 12 grams of protein in two eggs is enough to increase satiety by up to 50 percent and subsequently reduce the amount of calories you'll consume at lunch by about 164 calories. In the study, when 152 overweight adults ate a two-egg breakfast daily for 2 months, they lost 65 percent more weight than did another group that consumed the same number of calories for breakfast, but ate much less protein.

Don't be so concerned about eggs' effect on your cholesterol: New research shows that eating a couple of eggs a day will not raise your cholesterol levels, as once previously believed. In fact, we've learned that most blood cholesterol is made by the body from dietary fat, not dietary cholesterol.

7: Turkey and Other Lean Meats
(Lean Steak, Chicken, and Fish)

 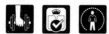

Superpowers: build muscle, improve the immune system

Secret weapons: protein, iron, zinc, creatine (beef), omega-3 fatty acids (fish), vitamins B6 (chicken and fish) and B12, phosphorus, potassium

Fight against: obesity, various diseases

Sidekicks: shellfish, Canadian bacon

Imposters: sausage, bacon, cured meats, ham, fatty cuts of steak such as T-bone and rib eye

A classic muscle-building nutrient, protein is the base of any solid diet plan. You already know that it takes more energy for your body to digest the protein in meat than it does to digest carbohydrates or fat, so the more protein you eat, the more calories you burn. Many studies support the notion that high-protein diets promote weight loss. In one study, researchers in Denmark found that people who substituted protein for 20 percent of their carbs were

||||||||||||||||||||||||||||||||||||||||||||||||||||||||||||||||||||||||||||||||||||||||||||||||||

Smart Substitutions

INSTEAD OF...	HAVE...	CALORIES SAVED
Sweet-and-sour pork	Beef with broccoli	480
8 jalapeño poppers	8 mozzarella sticks	345
Stuffed shells	Lasagna	295
Steak sandwich	Hamburger	208
Ham-and-cheese omelet	4 slices of bacon and 2 fried eggs	130
12-oz filet mignon	12-oz New York strip	120
Chocolate cake	Pecan pie	120
Turkey club (with mayo and bacon) with chips	Turkey dinner with mashed potatoes and stuffing	115

able to increase their metabolism and increase the number of calories they burned every day by up to 5 percent.

Among meats, turkey is a rare bird. Turkey breast is one of the leanest meats you'll find, and it packs nearly one-third of your daily requirements of niacin and vitamin B6. Dark meat, if you prefer, has lots of zinc and iron. One caution, though: If you're roasting a whole turkey for a family feast, avoid self-basting birds, which have been injected with fat.

Beef is another classic muscle-building protein. It's the top food source for creatine—the substance your body uses when you lift weights. Beef does have a downside; it contains saturated fats, but some cuts have more than others. Look for rounds or loins (that's code for extra-lean); sirloins and New York strips are less fatty than prime ribs and T-bones. Wash down that steak with a glass of fat-free milk. Research shows that calcium (that magic bullet again!) may reduce the amount of saturated fat your body absorbs. Choose cuts on the left side of the chart. They contain less fat but still pack high amounts of protein.

LEAN BEEF (55 calories and 2 to 3 grams of fat per 1-ounce serving)	MEDIUM-FAT BEEF (75 calories and 5 grams of fat per 1-ounce serving)
Flank steak	Corned beef
Ground beef (extra-lean or lean)	Ground beef (not marked as lean or extra-lean)
London broil	Prime cut
Roast beef	
Tenderloin	

To cut down on saturated fats even more, concentrate on fish like tuna and salmon, because they contain a healthy dose of omega-3 fatty acids as well as protein. Those fatty acids lower levels of a hormone called leptin in your body. Several recent studies suggest that leptin directly influences your metabolism: The higher your leptin levels, the more readily your body stores calories as fat. Researchers at the University of Wisconsin found that mice with low leptin levels have faster metabolisms and are able to burn fat faster than animals with higher leptin levels. Mayo Clinic researchers studying the diets of two African tribes found that the tribe that ate fish frequently had leptin levels nearly five

(continued on page 104)

What the Heck Is . . . Osteoporosis?

On the scale of strength, there's a big difference between the ends of the spectrum. There's the sturdy end—steel beams, diamonds, two-by-fours. And there's the fragile end—eggs, china, champagne flutes. Somewhere in between lies everything else. While it may seem that bones fall more toward the strong category, they're also very likely to swing toward the fragile side of the scale. While bones—which are actually living tissue that regenerates itself to form and build new bone cells throughout your life—are extremely strong (they're the second hardest substance in your body after enamel), your bone mass peaks at age 30. After that, your bones gradually get weaker and weaker, making them more porous, more fragile, and more prone to fractures.

Osteoporosis—a type of bone disease that comes from the thinning of bone tissue and loss of bone density—happens primarily to women because of their typically smaller bone mass (meaning it's quicker for women to feel the effects of more fragile bones), as well as hormonal factors. Women can lose up to 20 percent of their bone mass in the 5 to 7 years following menopause.

But the most important thing to know about osteoporosis and bone loss is that you can stop the decline by building new bone tissue and cells throughout your life. Many medications now help people who are most at risk of developing osteoporosis, and doctors advise getting a bone-density test as you reach menopause. (You don't notice any symptoms with osteoporosis, that is, until you break a bone.) But you can also do a number of other things to keep your skeleton strong. The Abs Diet serves as a great osteoporosis-prevention program, especially for its emphasis on both calcium and resistance training—two of the key components of basic bone building.

Drink more white stuff. And we're not talking liquefied icing. There's a reason why milk gets big play in magazine ads and billboards: It's one of the best sources of bone-building calcium. As you age, your body depletes calcium from your bones, leaving your skeleton deprived and more prone to thinning. Calcium—also found in other dairy products and some green, leafy vegetables like spinach—is the main mineral that helps build and maintain your skeletal structure. You need between 1,000 and 1,200 milligrams of calcium a day. You can get there with a couple of glasses of milk, a cup of yogurt, and a few slices of cheese.

Supplement it. If you're not sure you're getting enough dairy, you should consider taking a calcium supplement to make sure you're hitting the 1,200-milligram mark. Recent studies have shown that supplementing with a calcium pill can reduce the incidence of fractures by about 30 to 50 percent in people with low-calcium intakes.

Show some resistance. Studies have repeatedly shown that you need to include resistance training, like the kind found in the Abs Diet Workout, to help prevent bone loss. Penn State researchers even found that exercise is four times as effective as calcium for creating bone mass. In one University of Arizona study, women who did 20 to 25 minutes of resistance training and less than 10 minutes of cardiovascular weight-bearing activity, such as jogging or jumping rope, showed significant improvement in bone density. Weight-bearing exercise—like resistance training and running, as opposed to swimming or cycling, which doesn't require you to hold your own or additional weight—is what helps stimulate bones to grow. Even if you walk, it's important to include weight training for your upper body because walking can't help stimulate bone growth in your arms, shoulders, and wrists.

Add a D. As strong as it is, calcium alone can't help your bones. Your body needs vitamin D to help absorb it. Most people get enough because their skin absorbs it through sunlight, and there's plenty of D in the powerfoods (through the dairy products and fish, specifically). But as you get older, you may need to supplement with pills or D-fortified foods. Aim for between 200 and 400 IU daily.

Watch your protein. Here's another reason why excessively high protein diets are as harmful as chewing thumbtacks. Excessive amounts of protein can cause you to excrete calcium, forcing you to have a need for even greater amounts of calcium. As protein is burned for energy, it releases a substance called sulfate. High amounts mean that the sulfate starts increasing the excretion of calcium.

Use dumbbells. Do exercises that force you to balance yourself—that is, use dumbbells instead of weight-training machines and do abdominal work on a Swiss ball instead of the floor. Better balance won't help you build bone and prevent osteoporosis per se, but it will help prevent falls, which are the cause of many osteoporosis-related bone fractures.

times lower than the tribe that primarily ate vegetables. A bonus benefit for your fathers and husbands: Researchers in Stockholm studied the diets of more than 6,000 men and found that those who ate no fish had three times the risk of prostate cancer than those who ate it regularly. It's the omega-3s that inhibit prostate cancer growth.

Whether you eat fish or not, I want you to consider adding ground flaxseed to your food. As I pointed out earlier, 1 tablespoon contains only 60 calories, but it packs in omega-3 fatty acids and has nearly 4 grams of fiber. It has a nutty flavor, so you can sprinkle it into a lot of different recipes, add some to your meat or beans, spoon it over cereal, or add a tablespoon to a smoothie.

#8: Peanut Butter (All-Natural, Sugar-Free)

Superpowers: boosts testosterone, builds muscle, burns fat

Secret weapons: protein, monounsaturated fat, vitamin E, niacin, magnesium

Fights against: obesity, muscle loss, wrinkles, cardiovascular disease

Sidekicks: cashew and almond butters

Imposters: mass-produced sugary and trans fatty peanut butters

Yes, PB has its disadvantages: It's high in calories, and it doesn't go over well when you order it in four-star restaurants. But it's packed with those heart-healthy monounsaturated fats that can increase your body's production of testosterone, which can help your muscles grow and your fat melt. In one 18-month experiment, people who integrated peanut butter into their diets maintained weight loss better than those on low-fat plans. A recent study from the University of Illinois showed that diners who had monounsaturated fats before a meal (in this case, it was olive oil) ate 25 percent fewer calories during that meal than those who didn't.

Practically speaking, PB also works because it's a quick and versatile snack, and it tastes good. Because a diet that includes an indulgence like peanut butter doesn't leave you feeling deprived, it's easier to follow and won't make you fall prey to other cravings. Use it on an apple, on the go, or to add flavor to potentially bland smoothies. Two caveats: You can't gorge on it because of its fat content; limit yourself to just a couple tablespoons per day. And you should look for all-natural peanut butter, not the mass-produced brands that have added sugar.

#9: Olive Oil

Superpowers: lowers cholesterol, boosts the immune system

Secret weapons: monounsaturated fat, vitamin E

Fights against: obesity, cancer, heart disease, high blood pressure

Sidekicks: canola oil, peanut oil, sesame oil

Imposters: vegetable and hydrogenated vegetable oils, trans fatty acids, margarine

Olive oil and its brethren will help you eat less by controlling your food cravings; they'll also help you burn fat and keep your cholesterol in check. Do you need any more reason to pass the bottle?

#10: Whole-Grain Breads and Cereals

  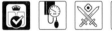

Superpower: prevent your body from storing fat

Secret weapons: fiber, protein, thiamin, riboflavin, niacin, pyridoxine, vitamin E, magnesium, zinc, potassium, iron, calcium

Fight against: obesity, cancer, high blood pressure, heart disease

Sidekicks: brown rice, whole-wheat pretzels, whole-wheat pastas

Imposters: processed bakery products such as white bread, bagels, and doughnuts; breads labeled wheat instead of whole wheat

There's only so long a person can survive on an all-protein diet or an all-salad diet or an all-anything diet. You will crave carbohydrates because your body needs carbohydrates. The key is to eat the ones that have been the least processed—carbs that still have all their heart-healthy, belly-busting fiber intact.

Whole-grain carbohydrates can play an important role in a healthy life-style. In an 11-year study of 16,000 middle-aged people, researchers at the University of Minnesota found that consuming three daily servings of whole grains can reduce a person's mortality risk over the course of a decade by 23 percent. (Tell that to your sister who's eating low-carb.) Whole-grain bread keeps insulin levels low, which keeps you from storing fat. In this diet, it's especially versatile because it'll supplement any kind of meal with little prep time. Toast for breakfast, sandwiches for lunch, with a dab of peanut butter for a snack. Don't believe the hype. Carbs—the right kind of carbs—are good for you.

Warning: Food manufacturers are very sneaky. Sometimes, after refining away all the vitamins, fiber, and minerals from wheat, they'll add molasses to the bread, turning it brown, and put it on the grocery shelf with a label that says wheat bread. It's a trick! Truly nutritious breads and other products will say "100 percent whole wheat" or "whole grain." Don't be fooled.

#11: Extra-Protein (Whey) Powder

Superpowers: builds muscle, burns fat

Secret weapons: protein, cysteine, glutathione

Fights against: obesity

Sidekick: ricotta cheese

Imposter: soy protein

Protein powder? What the heck is that? It's the only Abs Diet Power-food that you may not be able to find at the supermarket, but it's the one that's worth the trip to a health food store. I'm talking about powdered whey protein, a type of animal protein that packs a muscle-building wallop. If you add whey powder to your meal—in a smoothie, for instance—you may very well have created the most powerful fat-burning meal possible. Whey protein is a high-quality protein that contains essential amino acids that build muscle and burn fat. But it's especially effective because it has the highest amount of protein for the fewest number of calories, making it fat's

||||||||||||||||||||||||||||||||||||||||||||||||||||||||||||||||||||||||||||||||||||||||||||

Fat Content of Meat (4 oz, raw, without skin or bone)

	TOTAL (G)	SATURATED (G)
Skinless chicken breast	1.41	0.37
Veal steak	2.45	0.74
Wild rabbit	2.63	0.78
Lean ground beef	4	1.50
Cured ham	4.68	1.56
Wild duck breast	4.82	1.50
Chicken drumstick	5.05	1.34
Lean pork tenderloin	5.06	1.79
Beef sirloin steak	5.15	2
Buffalo	5.44	2.31
Turkey leg	7.62	2.34
Turkey breast	7.96	2.17
Lean beef tenderloin	8.02	3
Lean pork chop	8.19	2.85
Porterhouse steak	8.58	3
Lean ground turkey	9.37	2.55
Veal breast meat	9.73	3.80
Rib-eye steak	18.03	7.30
T-bone steak	19.63	7.69
Ham	21.40	7.42
Pork belly	60.11	21.92
Cured pork	91.29	33.32

kryptonite. Smoothies with some whey powder can be most effective before a workout. A 2001 study at the University of Texas found that people who drank a shake containing amino acids and carbohydrates before working out increased their protein synthesis (their ability to build muscle) more than those who drank the same shake after exercising. Because exercise increases bloodflow to tissues, the theory goes that having whey protein in your system when you work out may lead to a greater uptake of amino acids—the building blocks of muscle—in your muscle.

By the way, the one great source of whey protein in your supermarket is ricotta cheese. Unlike other cheeses, which are made from milk curd, ricotta is made from the whey left over from making mozzarella and provolone cheese—a good reason to visit your local Italian eatery.

ABS DIET SUCCESS STORY

"I don't feel restricted. I don't have cravings. I feel satisfied and energized."

Name: Kimberly Mayne

Age: 30

Height: 5'1"

Starting weight: 114

3 weeks later: 104

Despite being religious about her exercise routine, Kimberly Mayne didn't lead a healthy lifestyle: Her diet was a mess. "I used to spend hours in the gym, only to come home and eat processed lunches and dinners," she says. Poor eating habits sabotaged her efforts in the gym and she actually gained weight. Frustrated, she picked up *The Abs Diet for Women* and resolved to throw out her frozen dinners and learn to use a spatula.

"I was thrilled to find that cooking healthy wasn't difficult or more expensive than eating prepackaged meals," Mayne says. "I loved the fact that most recipes in the book have eight ingredients or less. Now that I'm cooking, for the first time in my life, I'm eating a healthy bal-

#12: Raspberries and Other Berries

Superpowers: protect your heart; enhance eyesight; improve balance, coordination, and short-term memory; prevent cravings

Secret weapons: antioxidants, fiber, vitamin C, tannins (cranberries)

Fight against: heart disease, cancer, obesity

Sidekicks: most other fruits, especially apples and grapefruit

Imposters: jellies, most of which eliminate fiber and add sugar

Depending on your taste, any berry will do (except Crunch Berries). I like raspberries as much for their power as for their taste. They carry powerful levels of antioxidants, all-purpose compounds that help your body fight heart dis-

---

ance of protein, carbohydrates, and healthy fats. I've learned that not all calories are created equal."

Mayne also changed her exercise routine, adopting the Abs Diet circuits and incorporating interval workouts into her schedule. Her new exercise mantra is "go hard and fast."

Within the first three weeks on the Abs Diet, Mayne lost 10 pounds and she has been able to maintain her weight for two years since she first picked up the book.

"I don't feel restricted with this eating plan and don't have cravings. Instead, I feel satisfied and energized."

Mayne's success on the Abs Diet inspired her mother, Christine, to try the program as well. In just three months, Christine lost 20 pounds and dropped her dress size from 12 to size 4.

She was amazed to find that the diet travels well. She continued the eating and exercise plan during a month-long vacation in Europe without gaining an ounce. (That's even after succumbing to a few holiday-season indulgences!)

Others have been similarly inspired by Mayne's new energy and passion for cooking. "Friends are amazed when I tell them that the best part is I'm eating more than I ever have before," say Mayne. "I explain that the Abs Diet is a lifestyle, not a diet. You can feel satisfied, and never go hungry if you provide your body with the essential nutrients it needs. That's something I can commit to for life."

ease and cancer; the berries' flavonoids may also help your eyesight, balance, coordination, and short-term memory. One cup of raspberries packs 6 grams of fiber and more than half of your daily requirement of vitamin C.

Blueberries are also loaded with the soluble fiber that, like oatmeal, keeps you fuller longer. In fact, they're one of the most healthful foods you can eat. Blueberries beat out 39 other fruits and vegetables in the antioxidant power ratings. One study also found that rats that ate blueberries were more coordinated and smarter than rats that didn't.

Strawberries contain another valuable form of fiber called pectin (as do grapefruits, peaches, apples, and oranges). In a study from the *Journal of the American College of Nutrition*, subjects drank plain orange juice or juice spiked with pectin. The people who got the loaded juice felt fuller after drinking it than those who got the juice without the pectin. The difference lasted for an impressive 4 hours.

Chapter 9

ABS DIET DISHES
Using Powerfoods in Quick and Easy Recipes

I
F YOU'RE LIKE A LOT OF people I work with and a lot of people I know, you spend more time in the bathroom, in the car, or on the couch than you do in the kitchen. You simply don't have time or the desire to cook. You grab breakfast on your way out; fill up on coffee when you get there; eat lunch with coworkers, clients, or kids; and swing by the vending machine or drive-thru in the afternoon. By the time you get home, the last thing you feel like doing is cooking.

Look, I was exactly the same way. My stove top was more likely to be littered with bills and junk mail than pots and pans. My oven used to be for storing stuff, not for roasting stuff. (Once, my mom came for a visit and accidentally baked my basketball.) The first time I cooked dinner for a girlfriend, she accurately identified the meal as "some kind of meat."

But that was before I realized how incredibly useful making your own meals can be for keeping weight off. By taking control in your kitchen, you can avoid eating the oversized, fat- and calorie-laden meals that restaurants typically serve up—foods that are making Americans obese in record numbers. Now, I've learned to cook and do it quickly and easily because even though I've recognized the power of making meals at home, I still don't have hours to devote to cooking. I'm sure you're the same way. So what you're going to see on the next few pages are recipes that can be made without having a degree from from the Culinary Institute of America. If you can operate a blender and a frying pan, you can handle these dishes.

Most of these recipes are ones you can make quickly—some in less than 5 minutes. I also know that you're not going to make every meal, so I've included sample combinations of foods that make properly balanced meals, utilizing the Abs Diet Powerfoods. For the dinners, serving sizes are often larger than one, so you can also use the leftovers for lunch. And if you've got a family to cook for, it's easy to double or even triple the recipes.

Abs Diet Smoothies

SMOOTHIES ARE ONE of the best parts about being on the Abs Diet. They take less than 3 minutes to make. They pack in multiple high-nutrient foods. They fill you up. If that's not enough, they can also taste like a five-star dessert. You can come up with your own concoctions by using 1 percent milk, low-fat vanilla yogurt, whey powder, and ice as the main ingredients. Oatmeal and fruit make nice additions, as does a spoonful of peanut butter. Include all ingredients in a blender and blend until smooth. For extra volume, add more ice. Here are some examples.

▶ FROM THE NEW ABS DIET COOKBOOK!

The Kitchen Sink (number of powerfoods: 6)

1 cup low-fat plain yogurt	1 teaspoons ground flaxseed
1 cup ice cubes	1 cup frozen strawberries or blueberries
¾ cup Fiber One cereal	
1 scoop vanilla whey protein	1 handful fresh baby spinach

Makes: 1½ servings

Per serving: 310 calories, 21 g protein, 29 g carbohydrates, 10 g fat (4 g saturated), 220 mg sodium, 19 g fiber

Abs Diet Ultimate Power Smoothie (number of powerfoods: 5)

1 cup 1 percent milk	**2** teaspoons peanut butter
2 tablespoons low-fat vanilla yogurt	**2** teaspoons chocolate whey powder
¾ cup instant oatmeal, nuked in water	**6** ice cubes, crushed

Makes: 2 8-ounce servings

Per serving: 220 calories, 12 g protein, 29 g carbohydrates, 4 g fat (1.5 g saturated), 118 mg sodium, 3 g fiber

▶ FROM THE NEW ABS DIET COOKBOOK!

Banana Split Smoothie (number of powerfoods: 3)

1 banana	**½** cup 1 percent milk
½ cup low-fat vanilla yogurt	**2** teaspoons whey powder
⅛ cup frozen orange juice concentrate	**6** ice cubes, crushed

Makes: 2 8-ounce servings

Per serving: 171 calories, 8 g protein, 33 g carbohydrates, 2 g fat (1 g saturated), 94 mg sodium, 2 g fiber

Halle Berries Smoothie (number of powerfoods: 4)

¾ cup instant oatmeal, nuked in water or fat-free milk	**2** teaspoons whey powder
¾ cup fat-free milk	**3** ice cubes, crushed
¾ cup mixed frozen blueberries, strawberries, and raspberries	(For a sweeter smoothie, add honey to taste.)

Makes: 2 8-ounce servings

Per serving: 144 calories, 7 g protein, 27 g carbohydrates, 1 g fat (0 g saturated), 109 mg sodium, 4 g fiber

PB&J Smoothie (number of powerfoods: 5)

$\frac{3}{4}$ cup low-fat vanilla yogurt

$\frac{3}{4}$ cup 1 percent milk

2 teaspoons peanut butter

1 medium banana

$\frac{1}{2}$ cup frozen unsweetened strawberries

2 teaspoons whey powder

4 ice cubes, crushed

Makes: 2 8-ounce servings

Per serving: 235 calories, 11 g protein, 39 g carbohydrates, 5 g fat (2 g saturated), 154 mg sodium, 4 g fiber

Summer Smoothie (number of powerfoods: 4)

$\frac{2}{3}$ cup frozen strawberries

1 banana

$\frac{1}{2}$ cup cubed honeydew melon

4 ounces low-fat vanilla yogurt

$\frac{3}{4}$ cup 1 percent milk

2 teaspoons vanilla whey powder

3 ice cubes, crushed

Makes: 2 8-ounce servings

Per serving: 199 calories, 9 g protein, 39 g carbohydrates, 2 g fat (1 g saturated), 117 mg sodium, 4 g fiber

▶ FROM THE NEW ABS DIET COOKBOOK!

Chocolate Pudding Milk Shake (number of powerfoods: 1)

3 cups cold nonfat milk

1 package (4 servings) Jell-O instant sugar-free chocolate pudding mix

$1\frac{1}{2}$ cups vanilla ice creamt

Makes: 5 servings

Per serving: 190 calories, 8 g protein, 31 g carbohydrates, 4.5 g fat (3 g saturated), 650 mg sodium, 2 g fiber

Belly-Busting Berry (number of powerfoods: 6)

1 scoop low-fat vanilla ice cream	1 tablespoon vanilla whey protein powder
¼ cup each frozen blueberries, strawberries, and raspberries	3 ice cubes
½ cup low-fat milk	

Makes: 1 8-ounce serving

Per serving: 251 calories, 15 g protein, 38 g carbohydrates, 4 g fat (2 g saturated), 116 mg sodium, 4 g fiber

Show Me the Honey (number of powerfoods: 3)

1 scoop low-fat butter pecan ice cream	1 teaspoon ground flaxseed
	1 dash cinnamon
½ cup low-fat milk	1 teaspoon honey
1 tablespoon vanilla whey protein powder	3 ice cubes

Makes: 1 8-ounce serving

Per serving: 250 calories, 15 g protein, 38 g carbohydrates, 4 g fat (2 g saturated), 131 mg sodium, 3 g fiber

Extreme Chocolate (number of powerfoods: 3)

1 scoop low-fat chocolate ice cream	1 tablespoon chocolate whey protein powder
1 tablespoon chocolate syrup	½ banana
½ cup low-fat chocolate milk	3 ice cubes

Makes: 1 8-ounce serving

Per serving: 355 calories, 17 g protein, 60 g carbohydrates, 6 g fat (4 g saturated), 158 mg sodium, 4 g fiber

The Orangeman (number of powerfoods: 3)

1 cup 1 percent milk	1 banana
½ cup frozen orange juice concentrate	2 teaspoons whey protein powder
2 tablespoons low-fat plain yogurt	6 ice cubes

Makes: 2 servings

Per serving: 241 calories, 10 g protein, 48 g carbohydrates, 2 g fat (1 g saturated), 84 mg sodium, 2 g fiber

▶ FROM THE NEW ABS DIET COOKBOOK!

Mango Tango (number of powerfoods: 4)

½ cup cubed mango	½ cup low-fat vanillla yogurt
⅓ cup blueberries	2 teaspoons vanilla whey protein powder
½ banana	
½ cup 1 percent milk	3 ice cubes

Makes: 2 servings

Per serving: 158 calories, 8 g protein, 29 g carbohydrates, 2 g fat (1 g saturated), 80 mg sodium, 2 g fiber

Lemon Drips and Drops (number of powerfoods: 5)

1 scoop low-fat vanilla ice cream	1 tablespoon vanilla whey protein powder
½ cup reduced-fat ricotta cheese	1 tablespoon sliced almonds
½ cup low-fat milk	½ lemon, juiced and zested
	3 ice cubes

Makes: 1 8-ounce serving

Per serving: 387 calories, 27 g protein, 37 g carbohydrates, 16 g fat (8 g saturated), 289 mg sodium, 2 g fiber

Abs Diet Breakfasts

BETWEEN GETTING A shower, skimming the paper, and the last-minute gluing you need to do on Bub's science fair project, breakfast is the martyr meal of the day. You usually sacrifice it for anything else that needs your attention. But if you had to rank the six meals in order of importance, the first meal would rank first. Breakfast wakes up your metabolism and tells it to start burning fat, decreasing your risk of obesity. The quickest way to incorporate the Abs Diet into your breakfast is to combine potent foods (specifically the Abs Diet Powerfoods) to make meals, such as:

▶ 8-ounce smoothie

▶ 2 tablespoons of peanut butter on whole-grain toast and 2 slices of Canadian bacon

▶ 1¾ cups of Shredded Wheat and Bran with 1 cup of 1 percent milk, 3 links of turkey sausage, and ½ cup of berries

▶ 2 scrambled eggs, 2 slices of whole-grain toast, 1 banana, and 1 cup of 1 percent or fat-free milk

▶ Cereal made with ¾ cup of high-fiber cereal, ¼ cup of Cap'n Crunch, 2 tablespoons of almonds, and ¾ cup of 1 percent or fat-free milk

▶ 1 slice of whole-grain bread with 1 tablespoon of peanut butter, 1 medium orange, ½ cup of All-Bran with ½ cup of 1 percent or fat-free milk and ½ cup of berries

▶ A hard-boiled egg, an apple, and 1 cup of low-fat chocolate milk

▶ A cheese stick and a small bag of homemade trail mix, including almonds, walnuts, raisins, dried cranberries and Cheerios

On the weekends or on mornings when you can spare a few more minutes, the breakfasts on the following pages will also deliver the appropriate nutritional punch.

▶ FROM THE NEW ABS DIET COOKBOOK!

Overtime Oats (number of powerfoods: 3)

4½ cups water	½ teaspoon salt
1 cup steel-cut oats	18 walnut halves
½ cup oat bran	2 large strawberries, sliced

1. Mix the water, oats, oat bran, and salt in a medium saucepan. Bring to a boil over medium-high heat. Reduce the heat and cover the pan. Simmer, stirring frequently, for 30 minutes or until thickened. Serve topped with the walnuts and strawberries.

Makes 3 1-cup servings

Per serving: 220 calories, 8 g protein, 31 g carbohydrates, 11 g fat (1.5 g saturated), 400 mg sodium, 6 g fiber

Eggs Beneficial Sandwich (number of powerfoods: 5)

1 large whole egg	1 slice Canadian bacon
3 large egg whites	1 tomato, sliced, or 1 green bell pepper, sliced
1 teaspoon ground flaxseed	
2 slices whole-wheat bread, toasted	½ cup orange juice

1. Scramble the whole egg and egg whites in a bowl. Add the ground flaxseed to the mixture.

2. Fry in a nonstick skillet spritzed with vegetable oil spray, and dump onto the toast.

3. Add the bacon and tomatoes, peppers, or other vegetables of your choice.

4. Drink the orange juice.

Makes: 1 serving

Per serving: 399 calories, 31 g protein, 46 g carbohydrates, 11 g fat (3 g saturated), 900 mg sodium, 6 g fiber

Breakfast Bacon Burger (number of powerfoods: 4)

1 Thomas' Honey Wheat English Muffin	1 slice low-fat American cheese
½ teaspoon trans fat–free margarine	1 slice Canadian bacon
1 egg	Vegetables of choice

1. Split the muffin, toast it, and spread it with the margarine.

2. Break the egg in a microwaveable dish, prick the yolk with a toothpick, and cover the dish with plastic wrap.

3. Microwave on high for 30 seconds. Let stand for 30 seconds. Add the cheese, egg, and Canadian bacon to the muffin, then nuke for 20 seconds.

4. Add vegetables to taste.

Makes: 1 serving

Per serving: 300 calories, 22 g protein, 28 g carbohydrates, 11 g fat (3.5 g saturated), 868 mg sodium, 3 g fiber

The I-Haven't-Had-My-Coffee-Yet Sandwich
(number of powerfoods: 3)

1½ teaspoons low-fat cream cheese	2 slices turkey or ham
1 whole-wheat pita, halved to make 2 pockets	Lettuce or green vegetable

1. Spread the cream cheese in the pockets of the pita.

2. Stuff with the meat and vegetables.

3. Put in mouth. Chew and swallow.

Makes: 1 serving

Per serving: 225 calories, 10 grams protein, 42 g carbohydrates, 3 g fat (1 g saturated), 430 mg sodium, 6 g fiber

▶ FROM THE NEW ABS DIET COOKBOOK!

Black Bean Breakfast Quesadillas (number of powerfoods: 5)

1 can (24 ounces) black beans, rinsed and drained

1 cup shredded, reduced-fat Monterey Jack cheese

1 jalapeño pepper, thinly sliced

8 whole-wheat tortillas

2 teaspoons olive oil

1 avocado, pitted, peeled and sliced

½ lime, cut into wedges

1. Preheat the oven to 200°F. Divide the beans, cheese, and peppers evenly among 4 tortillas. Top with the remaining tortillas.

2. Heat 1 teaspoon oil in a large nonstick skillet over medium-high heat. Put 2 quesadillas in the pan. Press down with a spatula as they cook. Shake the pan so they don't stick. Brown for 2 to 4 minutes, flip, and cook the other side until browned and the cheese is melted. Move the two finished quesadillas to the oven to keep warm. Then, repeat the process with the remaining oil and quesadillas.

3. Cut the quesadillas into quarters with a pizza cutter or knife. Top each quarter with 2 avocado slices. Squeeze lime juice on top.

Makes: 4 servings

Per serving: 460 calories, 20 g protein, 31 g carbohydrates, 11 g fat (1.5 g saturated), 400 mg sodium, 6g fiber

Mo' Feta, Mo' Betta (number of powerfoods: 3)

2 eggs

½ tablespoon feta cheese crumbles

⅓ cup torn baby spinach leaves

1 sprinkle dried oregano

In a microwave-safe bowl, mix the eggs until well blended. Add the feta, spinach, and oregano. Nuke for 2½ minutes, or until the eggs are set in the middle.

Makes: 1 serving

Per serving: 163 calories, 13 g protein, 2 g carbohydrates, 11 g fat (4 g saturated), 205 mg sodium, 0 g fiber

Waffles Rancheros (number of powerfoods: 2)

1 egg	1 tablespoon salsa
1 whole wheat toaster waffle	

Crack the egg in a small bowl, stir well until the yolk and white are well blended, and microwave for 2 minutes, 30 seconds. Prepare the waffle according to package directions. Top with the egg and salsa, cut in half, and stack.

Makes: *1 serving*

Per serving: *183 calories, 10 g protein, 14 g carbohydrates, 9 g fat (3 g saturated), 263 mg sodium, 1 g fiber*

Breakfast with Barbie (number of powerfoods: 3)

1 packet instant grits	1 tablespoon low-fat shredded Cheddar cheese
4 frozen shrimp, defrosted and chopped	1 dollop barbecue sauce

Prepare the grits according to package directions. Add the shrimp and cheese, stirring well to blend. Top with the barbecue sauce.

Makes: *1 serving*

Per serving: *167 calories, 9 g protein, 31 g carbohydrates, 1 g fat (0 g saturated), 731 mg sodium, 2 g fiber*

The 'Bama Bowl (number of powerfoods: 4)

1 packet instant grits	2 strips beef jerky, finely diced
1 teaspoon ground flaxseed	1 tablespoon low-fat shredded Cheddar cheese

Prepare the grits according to package directions. Add the flaxseed, jerky, and cheese, stirring well to blend.

Makes: *1 serving*

Per serving: *199 calories, 11 g protein; 26 g carbohydrates, 6 g fat (2 g saturated), 786 mg sodium, 3 g fiber*

Abs Diet Lunches

IN THE MIDDLE of the day, drive-throughs and pizza places can be more tempting than a hot tub at a ski resort. Be strong! You can still follow the eating plan no matter where you are. Grilled chicken and chili are usually good options. In sit-down situations, you can also order smartly without getting tripped up by the quesadilla special. Some good combinations include a salad with grilled chicken or salmon, vegetables, almonds or other nuts, and a sprinkling of balsamic vinegar and olive oil. You can also order a piece of lean meat—either on whole-grain bread or by itself—with a side of vegetables. Ask for salsa or a small side of olive oil for dipping. If you bring your lunch or eat it at home, these are some other options.

The I-Am-Not-Eating-Salad Salad (number of powerfoods: 4)

2 ounces grilled chicken

1 cup romaine lettuce

1 tomato, chopped

1 small green bell pepper, chopped

3 tablespoons 94 percent fat-free Italian dressing or 1 teaspoon olive oil

1 medium carrot, chopped

1 tablespoon grated Parmesan cheese

1 tablespoon ground flaxseed

1. Chop the chicken into small pieces.

2. Mix all the ingredients together and store in the fridge. Eat on multigrain bread or by itself.

Makes: 1 serving

Per serving: 248 calories, 16 g protein, 33 g carbohydrates, 8 g fat (2 g saturated), 875 mg sodium, 10 g fiber

Guilt-Free BLT (number of powerfoods: 3)

3/4 tablespoon fat-free mayonnaise

1 whole-wheat tortilla

2 slices turkey bacon, cooked

2 ounces roasted turkey breast, diced

2 slices tomato

2 leaves lettuce

1. Smear the mayo on the tortilla.

2. Line the middle of the tortilla with the bacon and top with turkey, tomato, and lettuce.

3. Roll it tightly into a tube.

Makes: 1 serving

Per serving: 206 calories, 17 g protein, 26 g carbohydrates, 7 g fat (2 g saturated), 1,270 mg sodium, 3 g fiber

Guac and Roll (number of powerfoods: 4)

1 can (6 ounces) light oil-packed tuna

2/3 cup guacamole

1/4 cup chopped tomatoes

1 teaspoon lemon juice

1 tablespoon light mayonnaise

1 teaspoon ground flaxseed

2 6-inch whole-wheat hoagie rolls

1. Combine the first six ingredients in a bowl and blend thoroughly with a fork.

2. Split the rolls in half and fill each half with 1/4 cup of the mixture.

Makes: 2 servings

Per serving: 606 calories, 36 g protein, 58 g carbohydrates, 28 g fat (5 g saturated), 942 mg sodium, 13 g fiber

Hot Tuna (number of powerfoods: 4)

½ cup chopped celery

1 onion, chopped

½ cup shredded, reduced-fat mozzarella cheese

½ cup reduced-fat cottage cheese

1 can (6 ounces) water-packed tuna, drained and flaked

¼ cup reduced-fat mayonnaise

1 tablespoon lemon juice

3 whole-wheat English muffins, split in half

1. Preheat your oven to 350°F. In a large nonstick skillet over low heat, cook the celery and onion until softened. Add the cheeses, tuna, mayo, and lemon juice to the skillet and cook the mixture just long enough to warm it up.

2. Spread ⅙ of the mixture on each English muffin half. Put the muffin halves on a baking sheet and bake for 10 minutes.

Makes: 2 servings

Per serving: 628 calories, 50 g protein, 54 g carbohydrates, 24 g fat (6 g saturated), 1,300 mg sodium, 8 g fiber

▶ FROM THE NEW ABS DIET COOKBOOK!

The Johnny Apple Cheese Sandwich (number of powerfoods: 3)

2 slices 7-grain bread

2 teaspoons light mayonnaise

1 teaspoon Dijon mustard

2 slices low-fat Swiss cheese

1 Red Delicious apple, halved and thinly sliced

1 tablespoon chopped walnuts

1. Preheat a toaster oven to 350°F.

2. Spread 1 bread slice with mayonnaise and the other with mustard. Top each with cheese.

3. Place on a tray and put into the toaster oven until the cheese has melted. Top 1 bread slice with the apple and sprinkle with the walnuts. Press the sandwich halves together.

Makes: 1 serving

Per serving: 440 calories, 19 g protein, 46 g carbohydrates, 21 g fat (7 g saturated), 500 mg sodium, 8 g fiber

Crunch Time (number of powerfoods: 5)

3 cups mixed greens

2 slices smoked deli turkey, chopped

½ small Granny Smith apple, chopped

2 tablespoons grated carrot

1 tablespoon diced pecans

1½ tablespoons Craisins (dried, sweetened cranberries)

1 tablespoon blue cheese crumbles

For dressing: 1½ teaspoons olive oil; 1 tablespoon balsamic vinegar

In a bowl, mix together all of the ingredients. Store in the fridge until you are ready to eat.

Makes: *1 serving*

Per serving: *296 calories, 15 g protein, 31 g carbohydrates, 15 g fat (3 g saturated), 590 mg sodium, 7 g fiber*

Hurry Curry (number of powerfoods: 3)

½ cup fat-free plain yogurt

½ cup fat-free mayonnaise

3 tablespoons finely chopped onion

1 teaspoon ginger

1 teaspoon curry powder

1 pound boneless, skinless chicken breasts, cut into ½-inch strips

1 teaspoon paprika

½ teaspoon ground black pepper

2 cups cooked brown rice

1. In a small bowl, mix the yogurt, mayonnaise, onion, ginger, and curry powder.

2. Place the chicken in a medium bowl. Sprinkle with the paprika and pepper. Toss until coated.

3. In a nonstick skillet over medium heat, cook the chicken for 4 to 5 minutes. Stir in the yogurt mixture. Cook, stirring, for 2 minutes. Serve over the rice.

Makes: *2 servings*

Per serving: *598 calories, 61 g protein, 69 g carbohydrates, 7 g fat (1 g saturated), 704 mg sodium, 6 g fiber*

▶ **FROM THE NEW ABS DIET COOKBOOK!**

Man-Can-Live-Without-Bread Chicken Salad Sandwich
(number of powerfoods: 2)

2 cooked chicken breast
halves, chopped

½ cup chopped celery

½ scallion, chopped

2 tablespoons light
mayonnaise

Salt and pepper

½ cup halved seedless red grapes

2 romaine or red leaf lettuce
leaves

1. Mix the chicken, celery, scallion, and mayonnaise in a bowl; season with salt and pepper. Gently stir in the grapes.

2. Divide between the lettuce leaves and roll up.

Makes 2 servings

Per serving: 230 calories, 27 g protein, 10 g carbohydrates, 8 g fat (1.5 g saturated), 200 mg sodium, 1 g fiber

Roll of a Lifetime (number of powerfoods: 4)

¾ cup diced precooked
chicken

2 tablespoons diced onion

2 tablespoons feta cheese
crumbles

1 handful romaine lettuce,
chopped

1 large whole wheat tortilla

Salsa for dipping

1. Arrange the chicken, onion, cheese, and lettuce down the center of the tortilla.

2. Roll tightly, then cut in half.

3. Place the rolls seam side down on a nonstick skillet heated to medium heat. Grill for 2 to 3 minutes per side. Serve with the salsa.

Makes: 1 serving

Per serving: 397 calories, 56 g protein, 25 g carbohydrates, 10 g fat (4 g saturated), 493 mg sodium, 3 g fiber

Popeye and Olive Oil (number of powerfoods: 4)

1½ cups chopped baby spinach leaves

1½ cups chopped romaine lettuce

3 slices prosciutto, chopped

⅓ cup mandarin orange slices

⅓ cup sliced strawberries

2 tablespoons diced red onion

For dressing: 1½ teaspoons olive oil; 1 tablespoon red wine vinegar; ½ clove garlic, crushed; ⅛ teaspoon black pepper

In a bowl, mix together all of the ingredients. Store in the fridge until you are ready to eat.

Makes: *1 serving*

Per serving: *238 calories, 9 g protein, 23 g carbohydrates, 14 g fat (4 g saturated), 450 mg sodium, 6 g fiber*

Reuben Reduced (number of powerfoods: 5)

¼ cup canned sauerkraut, drained

1 tablespoon feta cheese crumbles

1 tablespoon low-fat Thousand Island dressing

2 slices rye bread

2 slices reduced-sodium smoked deli turkey, such as Healthy Choice

1 slice low-fat Swiss cheese

1. Coat the bottom of a nonstick skillet with cooking spray and heat over medium heat.

2. In a small bowl, stir together the kraut, feta, and dressing. Spread on one slice of the bread. Top with the turkey, Swiss, and remaining slice of bread.

3. Grill for 2 to 3 minutes per side.

Makes: *1 serving*

Per serving: *335 calories, 23 g protein, 42 g carbohydrates, 9 g fat (3 g saturated), 1,625 mg sodium, 5 g fiber*

The Melon Banquet (number of powerfoods: 4)

3 cups mixed greens	**1** tablespoon pine nuts
⅓ cup cubed watermelon	**1** teaspoon chopped mint
½ cup cubed cantaloupe	**For dressing:**
2 tablespoons grated carrot	**1½** teaspoons olive oil
1 ounce smoked salmon, chopped	**2** teaspoons balsamic vinegar;
	1 teaspoon lemon juice

In a bowl, mix together all of the ingredients. Store in the fridge until you are ready to eat.

Makes: 1 serving

Per serving: 274 calories, 11 g protein, 20 g carbohydrates, 19 g fat (2 g saturated), 635 mg sodium, 5 g fiber

Drink This

SAVE LOADS OF calories by substituting unsweetened iced tea for sugary sodas. Or try this lightly sweet, low-calorie concoction.

The Abs Diet Arnold Palmer

7 cups water	**1** lime, sliced
2 black tea bags	**1** lemon, sliced
1 cup loosely packed mint leaves	**1** orange, sliced
1 can (6 ounces) frozen lemonade concentrate, thawed	

1. Boil 3 cups of the water. Add the tea bags and mint. Steep for 10 minutes.

2. Strain the tea into a 3-quart container. Stir in the remaining 4 cups water and lemonade. Add slices of lime, lemon, and orange as garnish. Serve in tall glasses over ice.

Makes: 8 servings

Per serving: 15 calories, 0 g protein, 5 g carbohydrates, 0 g fat, 5 mg sodium, 0 g fiber

Abs Diet Dinners

DINNER IS THE place where most of us wind down and pork up. That's because we spend the day serving others. By dinnertime, we're hungry to have some of our own demands met. On this plan, you'll have already fueled up four times before dinner, so you'll feel pleasantly hungry, not ravenous. These meals give you the taste of sin—without the actual guilt.

Italian Chowin' (number of powerfoods: 4)

1 pound extra-lean ground beef

½ cup crushed saltine crackers

1 large onion, diced

1 clove garlic, minced

1 tablespoon ground flaxseed or whey powder

1 jar (16 ounces) tomato sauce

4 whole-wheat hoagie rolls

½ cup reduced-fat mozzarella cheese, shredded

1. Mix the beef, crackers, onion, garlic, and flaxseed or whey powder into golf ball–size meatballs.

2. In a nonstick skillet over medium heat, cook the meatballs until browned all the way around. Drain the fat from the skillet and add the tomato sauce.

3. While the mixture is warming, use a fork to scoop out some of the bread in the rolls to form shallow trenches. Spoon the meatballs and sauce into each trench, sprinkle with the cheese, and top with the top half of the roll.

Makes: 4 servings

Per serving: 569 calories, 38 g protein, 65 g carbohydrates, 19 g fat (6 g saturated), 1,341 mg sodium, 10 g fiber

Brazilian Chicken (number of powerfoods: 2)

1 lemon

1 lime

1 tablespoon ground flaxseed

1 can (8 ounces) tomato sauce

1 can (6 ounces) frozen orange juice concentrate

1½ cloves garlic, minced

1 teaspoon dried Italian seasoning

1 teaspoon hot pepper salsa

4 boneless, skinless chicken breast halves

¾ cup chunky salsa

1. Grate the zest of the lemon and lime into a resealable bag. Squeeze the juice from both fruits into the bag and throw out the pulp and the seeds.

2. Mix in everything else except the chicken and chunky salsa.

3. Drop in the chicken, reseal the bag, and refrigerate for a few hours.

4. Grill the chicken, turning and basting with marinade a few times, for 10 to 15 minutes, or until the center is no longer pink. Serve with the salsa.

Makes: 4 servings

Per serving: 205 calories, 29 g protein, 18 g carbohydrates, 2 g fat (0.5 g saturated), 726 mg sodium, 3 g fiber

▶ FROM THE NEW ABS DIET COOKBOOK!

Maria's Portobellos (number of powerfoods: 1)

2 tablespoons extra-virgin olive oil

2 tablespoons balsamic vinegar

1 clove garlic, minced

1 pound large portobello mushrooms

Salt and pepper

Mix the oil, vinegar, and garlic in a large bowl. Add the mushrooms and gently toss to coat. Allow the mushrooms to marinate for 30 minutes. Remove from the marinade and grill, roast, or broil until golden brown. Season with salt and pepper.

Makes: 6 servings

Per serving: 70 calories, 2 g protein, 5 g carbohydrates, 5 g fat (0.5 g saturated), 200 mg sodium, 1 g fiber

Chili Con Turkey (number of powerfoods: 4)

1 pound ground turkey

1 can (14 ounces) Mexican-style diced tomatoes

1 can (15 ounces) black beans, rinsed and drained

1 can (14 ounces) whole-kernel sweet corn, drained

1 package (1½ ounces) dried chili mix

1 tablespoon ground flaxseed

¼ cup water

1 cup cooked brown rice

1. In a large nonstick skillet over medium-high heat, brown the turkey.

2. Add everything else but the rice and cook over low heat for 10 minutes. Serve over the rice.

Makes: *4 servings*

Per serving: *407 calories, 30 g protein, 52 g carbohydrates, 11 g fat (3 g saturated), 1,578 mg sodium, 9 g fiber*

Chicken à la King Kong (number of powerfoods: 3)

2 tablespoons olive oil

½ onion, finely chopped

1 teaspoon flour

2 tablespoons water

1 pound chicken breast tenders

4 teaspoons chili powder

1 cup spaghetti sauce

9 ounces cooked whole-wheat spaghetti

1. Heat the oil in a nonstick skillet over medium-high heat. Add the onion and cook for 1 minute, until browned. In a small bowl, mix the flour and water.

2. Add the chicken, chili powder, sauce, and flour mixture to the skillet. Stir. Simmer uncovered for 10 minutes. Serve over the spaghetti.

Makes: *4 servings*

Per serving: *320 calories, 31 g protein, 26 g carbohydrates, 10 g fat (2 g saturated), 360 mg sodium, 5 g fiber*

Salmon Rushdie (number of powerfoods: 5)

2	tablespoons olive oil	1	clove garlic
1	tablespoon lemon juice	4	salmon fillets (6 ounces each)
¼	teaspoon salt		Green vegetable of choice
¼	teaspoon ground black pepper	1	cup cooked brown rice
1	tablespoon ground flaxseed		

1. In a baking dish, combine the oil, lemon juice, salt, pepper, flaxseed, and garlic. Add the fish, coat well, cover, and refrigerate for 15 minutes.

2. Preheat your oven to 450°F. Line a baking sheet with foil and coat it with cooking spray. Remove the fish from the marinade and place the fish skin side down on the baking sheet.

3. Bake for 9 to 12 minutes. Serve with a green vegetable and the rice.

Makes: 4 servings

Per serving: 411 calories, 40 g protein, 15 g carbohydrates, 20 g fat (3 g saturated), 231 mg sodium, 1 g fiber

BBQ King (number of powerfoods: 5)

5	ounces smoked turkey kielbasa, diced	1	can (14½ ounces) pureed tomatoes
1	small onion, chopped		Salt and pepper
1	can (3 ounces) sliced mushrooms	¼	cup seasoned bread crumbs
1	clove garlic, minced	¾	tablespoon ground flaxseed
1	can (16 ounces) baked beans	¾	tablespoon olive oil
1	can (8 ounces) navy beans, drained		

1. Preheat your oven to 350°F. Put the kielbasa in a 2-quart baking dish and bake until browned (about 5 minutes). Drain the fat and set the dish aside.

2. In a nonstick skillet over medium-high heat, cook the onion, mushrooms, and garlic for 5 to 7 minutes. Transfer to the baking dish, then add the beans and tomatoes, plus salt and pepper to taste.

3. Bake for 20 minutes or until the edges bubble.

4. In a small bowl, mix the bread crumbs and flaxseed with the oil. Sprinkle over the sausage mixture and broil 4 to 5 inches from the heat, until the top is golden (about 3 minutes).

Makes: *4 servings*

Per serving: *348 calories, 20 g protein, 53 g carbohydrates, 8.5 g fat (2 g saturated), 1,463 mg sodium, 13 g fiber*

Spaghettaboudit! (number of powerfoods: 3)

¾ pound extra-lean ground beef

1½ onions, chopped

1 green bell pepper, chopped

2 cloves garlic, minced

1 cup sliced mushrooms

2 cans (16 ounces) whole tomatoes

1 jar (20 ounces) spaghetti sauce

2 tablespoons Italian seasoning

1 package (1 pound) whole-wheat spaghetti

1. In a large saucepan over medium-high heat, cook the meat until browned. Drain the fat from the meat.

2. Add the onions, pepper, and garlic, and cook until tender. Pour in the mushrooms, tomatoes (with juice), sauce, and seasoning, and stir everything together. Simmer. In a separate pot, cook the spaghetti according to the package directions.

3. Serve ½ cup of the sauce over 1 cup of the spaghetti.

Makes: *4 servings*

Per serving: *400 calories, 28 g protein, 50 g carbohydrates, 12 g fat (4 g saturated), 798 mg sodium, 10 g fiber*

▶ **FROM THE NEW ABS DIET COOKBOOK!**

A Thinner Mexican Dinner (number of powerfoods: 5)

For the meat:

- ¾ pound lean ground beef (90 percent lean or higher)
- 2 cloves garlic, minced
- 1 can (15.5 ounces) black beans, rinsed and drained
- 1 tablespoon chili powder
- ¼ teaspoon cayenne
- ⅓ cup water

For the dressing:

- 4 medium tomatoes, diced
- 2 tablespoons extra-virgin olive oil
- 2 tablespoons lime juice
- ½ teaspoon salt
- ¼ teaspoon black pepper

For the salad:

- 2 romaine lettuce hearts, chopped
- ½ cup shredded reduced-fat Cheddar cheese
- 2 ounces baked corn tortilla chips (about 32 chips)

1. Heat a large skillet over medium-high heat. Add the beef and cook, breaking up the pieces with a wooden spoon, until no longer pink. Add the garlic and beans and cook for 2 minutes more. Add the chili powder, cayenne, and water and stir until well combined and some but not all of the liquid has been absorbed. Remove from the heat and allow the mixture to cool slightly.

2. Mix the dressing ingredients in a bowl.

3. Divide the lettuce among dinner plates, top with the beef mixture, and sprinkle with cheese. Spoon the dressing over each salad and crush tortilla chips on top.

Makes: 4 servings

Per serving: 440 calories, 32 g protein, 43 g carbohydrates, 19 g fat (6 g saturated), 870 mg sodium, 11 g fiber

Gone Fishing (number of powerfoods: 5)

1 tablespoon + 1 teaspoon olive oil

1 trout fillet

1 tablespoon cornmeal

Salt and pepper

½ teaspoon chopped fresh parsley

1 cup French green beans, trimmed and cut into bite-size pieces

2 teaspoons sliced almonds

1. Heat 1 tablespoon of the oil in a nonstick skillet over medium heat.

2. While the pan is heating, sprinkle the flesh side of the trout with the cornmeal, salt, and pepper, pressing lightly so the cornmeal sticks.

3. Place in the pan, flesh side down, and sauté for 4 minutes. Flip and cook for another 2 minutes. Top with the parsley.

4. Place the beans into a steamer basket and steam for 5 minutes. Toss with the remaining 1 teaspoon oil, almonds, salt, and pepper.

Makes: *1 serving*

Per serving: *372 calories, 20 g protein, 17 g carbohydrates, 26 g fat (4 g saturated), 48 mg sodium, 5 g fiber*

Terra Ricotta (number of powerfoods: 3)

3 tablespoons reduced-fat ricotta cheese

1 teaspoon ready-made roasted garlic

1 ready-made flatbread, such as Flat Out

¾ cup chopped precooked chicken

3 tablespoons grated reduced-fat mozzarella cheese

Salt and pepper

Stir together the ricotta and garlic, blending well. Spread on the flatbread. Top with the chicken and mozzarella. Season to taste with salt and pepper. Bake at 375°F for 6 minutes.

Makes: *1 serving*

Per serving: *352 calories, 41 g protein, 19 g carbohydrates, 13 g fat (6 g saturated), 409 mg sodium, 2 g fiber*

▶ FROM THE NEW ABS DIET COOKBOOK!

Yes, You Can Grill Caesar Salad (number of powerfoods: 3)

- 1 French baguette
- 2 tablespoons extra-virgin olive oil
- ⅓ cup light mayonnaise
- ¼ cup grated Parmesan cheese
- 3 tablespoons lemon juice
- 1 teaspoon anchovy paste
- ¼ teaspoon black pepper
- 1 clove garlic, halved
- 1 package romaine lettuce hearts

1. Cut the bread into ½-inch slices. Brush both sides of the slices lightly with oil. Grill over medium heat for 3 minutes per side to toast. Set aside to cool.

2. Mix the mayonnaise, cheese, lemon juice, anchovy paste, pepper, and any remaining oil in a large bowl until smooth; refrigerate until needed.

3. Rub the cut garlic over both sides of each bread slice. Cut the bread into ½-inch cubes to make the croutons.

4. Cut each head of the romaine lettuce in half lengthwise. Grill about 5 minutes or until wilted and slightly browned on each side, turning once. Place each half on a salad plate, drizzle with the dressing, and toss on the croutons. Finish with a sprinkle of cheese.

Makes: 4 servings

Per serving: 245 calories, 7 g protein, 20 g carbohydrates, 14 g fat (3 g saturated), 420 mg sodium, 3 g fiber

Colonel Mustard (number of powerfoods: 3)

1 tablespoon maple syrup	2 thin-cut boneless pork chops
1 tablespoon Dijon mustard	2 cups Italian salad greens
1 teaspoon olive oil	1 tablespoon low-fat balsamic vinaigrette
Salt and pepper	

1. In a small bowl, stir together the syrup, mustard, oil, salt, and pepper until well blended.

2. Place the chops and mustard mixture inside a large zip-top plastic bag, then shake to coat the chops.

3. Place the chops on a nonstick skillet heated to medium-high, cooking 2 to 3 minutes per side. In the last minute of cooking, pour the remaining mustard mixture onto the chops as they cook.

4. Toss the greens and dressing in a large bowl to coat.

Makes: 1 serving

Per serving: 393 calories, 42 g protein, 23 g carbohydrates, 17 g fat (5 g saturated), 650 mg sodium, 2 g fiber

The Orange and Gold (number of powerfoods: 5)

2 teaspoons peanut oil	1/3 cup chopped celery
1/4 teaspoon red-pepper flakes	1 green onion, sliced
2 thin-cut boneless, skinless chicken breasts, cut into bite-size pieces or strips	2 tablespoons chopped unsalted roasted peanuts
1/3 cup matchstick carrots	1 tablespoon hoisin sauce

1. Combine the oil and pepper flakes in a medium-hot skillet.

2. Add the chicken and cook for 2 to 3 minutes, stirring frequently.

3. Add the remaining ingredients and cook for 2 to 3 minutes, stirring frequently. Serve over brown rice.

Makes: 1 serving

Per serving: 356 calories, 45 g protein, 18 g carbohydrates, 11 g fat (2 g saturated), 444 mg sodium, 5 g fiber

Chicken Little Italy (number of powerfoods: 3)

1 tablespoon + 1 teaspoon olive oil	1 teaspoon Parmesan cheese
	Salt and pepper to taste
1 boneless, skinless chicken breast	¼ cup spaghetti sauce
1 tablespoon Italian-seasoned bread crumbs	1 small clove garlic, crushed
	3 handfuls baby spinach leaves

1. Heat 1 tablespoon of the oil in a nonstick skillet over medium heat.

2. While the pan is heating, pound the chicken to ¼-inch thickness, then sprinkle with the bread crumbs, cheese, salt, and pepper, pressing lightly so the crumbs stick.

3. Place in the pan and sauté for 2 to 3 minutes per side. Top with nuked spaghetti sauce.

4. Combine the remaining 1 teaspoon oil and the garlic in another nonstick skillet over medium-high heat.

5. Add the spinach, turning frequently with tongs until wilted (about 6 minutes).

Makes: 1 serving

Per serving: 395 calories, 32 g protein, 19 g carbohydrates, 22 g fat (3 g saturated), 608 mg sodium, 5 g fiber

▶ FROM THE NEW ABS DIET COOKBOOK!

The Weight-Loss Burger (number of Abs Diet powerfoods: 4)

10 ounces ground buffalo, divided into two patties	4 large romaine lettuce leaves, ribs removed
1 teaspoon extra-virgin olive oil	⅓ cup shredded sharp Cheddar cheese
Salt and pepper	
2 slices red onion	Ketchup
2 eggs	Dijon mustard

1. Form the meat into 2 patties. For medium-rare burgers, allow the meat to rest at room temperature for about 30 minutes. Brush with the oil and season with salt and pepper.

2. Grill over high heat for 4 minutes per side. At the same time, grill the onion slices until lightly charred.

3. Fry the eggs in a nonstick skillet until the desired degree of doneness.

4. Cut carbs by going bun-free: For each serving, overlap 2 lettuce leaves on a plate, top with the burger, fried egg, cheese, onion, ketchup, and mustard. Fold the lettuce over the burger and eat with both hands.

Makes: 2 servings

Per serving: 370 calories, 7 g protein, 19 g carbohydrates, 19 g fat (8 g saturated), 450 mg sodium, 1 g fiber

Abs Diet Snacks

MOST DIET PLANS portray snacking as a failure. I want you to think of snacking as exactly the opposite—as a key to success! But the secret to effective snacking is doing so at the optimum time—about 2 hours before you're scheduled to eat your next meal. That'll be enough time to head off hunger pangs and keep you full enough to avoid a meltdown at mealtime. You have a lot of flexibility in what you use to snack. You could use one of the recipes that follow or have a portion of leftovers from dinner, a sandwich, a smoothie, or a combination of some of the Abs Diet Powerfoods. To make it easier, pick one food from column A and one from column B below. That will ensure your satiety.

A		B	
PROTEIN	**DAIRY**	**FRUIT OR VEGETABLE**	**COMPLEX CARBOHYDRATE**
2 teaspoons reduced-fat peanut butter	8 ounces low-fat yogurt	1 ounce raisins	1 or 2 slices whole-grain bread
1 ounce almonds	1 cup 1 percent milk or chocolate milk	Raw vegetables (celery, baby carrots, broccoli), unlimited	1 bowl oatmeal or high-fiber cereal
3 slices low-sodium deli turkey breast	¾ cup low-fat ice cream	1½ cups berries	
3 slices deli roast beef	1½ slices fat-free cheese	4 ounces cantaloupe	
	1 stick string cheese	1 large orange	
		1 can (11.5 ounces) low-sodium V8 juice	

Cucumber Tubes (number of powerfoods: 5)

1 cucumber

1 teaspoon finely chopped parsley

¼ teaspoon finely chopped basil

½ teaspoon finely chopped chives

¾ cup low-fat, low-sodium cottage cheese

Cut the cucumber in half lengthwise. Hollow the center of each half by scooping out the seeds with a spoon or vegetable knife. Stir the herbs into the cottage cheese, then arrange in the hollowed cucumbers.

Makes: 2 servings

Per serving: 84 calories, 12 g protein, 7 g carbohydrates, 1 g fat (1 g saturated), 11 mg sodium, 2 g fiber

PB Power Apples (number of powerfoods: 2)

2 tablespoons peanut butter

Dash of cinnamon

1 medium red apple, such as Gala or Red Delicious, halved and cored

In a small bowl, stir together the peanut butter and cinnamon (start with a dash—cinnamon is potent stuff). Spread on each apple half.

Makes: 1 serving

Per serving: 276 calories, 8 g protein, 30 g carbohydrates, 17 g fat (3 g saturated), 1 mg sodium, 8 g fiber

Spread Yourself Thin (number of powerfoods: 2)

1 can (15 ounces) cannellini beans, rinsed and drained

1 tablespoon chopped fresh rosemary

1 clove garlic, crushed

½ lemon, juiced

2 tablespoons olive oil

Salt and pepper

In a blender or food processor, mix the beans, rosemary, garlic, and lemon juice. (If you're using a blender, you may need to stop and scrape the sides of the canister once to make sure everything blends well.) Stream the oil through the top until you reach the desired consistency. Season to taste with salt and pepper.

Per 1-tablespoon serving: 21 calories, 1 g protein, 2 g carbohydrates, 1 g fat (0 g saturated), 20 mg sodium, 1 g fiber

Yogi Pops (number of powerfoods: 1)

1 6-pack (4-ounce cups) of your favorite flavor of reduced-fat yogurt

6 Popsicle sticks

Pierce each yogurt pack with a stick. Freeze.

Makes: 6 servings

Per serving: 118 calories, 4 g protein, 24 g carbohydrates, 1 g fat (0 g saturated), 59 mg sodium, 0 g fiber

|||||||||||||||||||||||||||||||||||||||||||||||||||||||||||||||||||||||||||||||||||||||||||||||||||||||||||||

How to Pick a Better Yogurt

Shoot for more protein: Greek yogurt contains up to 18 grams of protein per serving (three times the amount in some regular yogurts).

Hunt for calcium: Choose a yogurt that contains at least 20 percent of your daily calcium needs.

Keep the calorie count around 100: Plain yogurt contains a relatively small amount of natural sugar and hovers around 100 calories. The sweeter flavored fruit yogurts can contain 170 calories per serving.

Make it better: If you want a sweeter yogurt, add a healthy sugar, like blueberries and raisins. Toss in some walnuts or almonds for added nutrition.

Chapter 10

ABS DIET MEAL PLANS
Featuring 3 Perfect Weeks
of Eating for Women

U NLIKE MOST DIET PLANS, which are laden with complex, hard-to-follow rules and verboten foods you love but have to live without, the Abs Diet lets you eat the foods you love, keeps your cravings at bay, and helps you control stress—all at the same time. Here's an example of how you can structure a week of eating. It's not written in stone, by any means: Mix up the meals. Substitute whenever you want. Heck, I don't care if you eat the same thing every day for a week. The purpose of these sample weeks are simply to show you how to follow the principles of the Abs Diet. So enjoy!

The calories in the weekly meal plans below are tailored to provide between 1,400 and 1,600 calories per day. But every woman has different caloric needs, depending on her current weight and activity level (page 69 gave you a formula to figure out yours). Use these weekly meal plans as a base, but you can also adjust either up or down. If you want to reduce your calories, don't skip a meal—remember, eating six times a day helps keep your metabolism moving. Instead, cut the portion size of a regular meal or eliminate part of a snack. If your formula shows that you should add calories, I recommend that you increase in small ways, such as drinking a few more ounces of smoothie for a meal or snack or adding a handful of nuts at a snack, rather than augmenting too much during your meals, where there's more chance of doling out larger-than-you-need portions.

Perfect Week, Sample 1

MONDAY: 1,250 CALORIES

Breakfast

Waffles Rancheros (page 121)

Snack #1

8 ounces Belly-Busting Berry smoothie (page 115), 1 apple

Lunch

Crunch Time (page 125), 1 stick string cheese

Snack #2

Cucumber Tubes (page 140)

Dinner

Gone Fishing (page 135)

Snack #3

Low-fat ice cream sandwich

TUESDAY: 1,420 CALORIES

Breakfast

Overtime Oats (page 117)

Snack #1

8 ounces Show Me the Honey smoothie (page 118)

Lunch

Roll of a Lifetime (page 126), 1 cup berries

Snack #2

1 stick string cheese, 5 to 7 whole-wheat crackers, such as Triscuits

Dinner

Terra Ricotta (page 135)

Snack #3

Yogi Pops (page 141)

WEDNESDAY: 1,355 CALORIES

Breakfast

Mo' Feta, Mo' Betta (page 120)

Snack #1

8 ounces Extreme Chocolate smoothie (page 115)

Lunch

Popeye and Olive Oil (page 127)

Snack #2

½ PB Power Apples (page 140)

Dinner

Colonel Mustard (page 137)

Snack #3

Low-fat ice cream sandwich

THURSDAY: 1,470 CALORIES

Breakfast

Waffles Rancheros (page 121), 1 pear

Snack #1

8 ounces Banana Split smoothie (page 113)

Lunch

Reuben Reduced (page 127)

Snack #2

1 stick string cheese, 5 to 7 whole-wheat crackers, such as Triscuits

Dinner

The Orange and Gold (page 137)

Snack #3

Yogi Pops (page 141)

FRIDAY: 1,300 CALORIES

Breakfast

Breakfast with Barbie (page 121)

Snack #1

8 ounces Chocolate Pudding Milk Shake smoothie (page 114)

Lunch

The Melon Banquet (page 128)

Snack #2

Cucumber Tubes (page 140)

Dinner

A Thinner Mexican Dinner (page 134)

Snack #3

1 carton low-fat yogurt with fruit

SATURDAY: 1,540 CALORIES

Breakfast

Black Bean Quesadillas, 1 orange (page 120)

Snack #1

8 ounces Belly-Busting Berry smoothie (page 115)

Lunch

Man Can Live Without Bread Chicken Salad (page 126)

Snack #2

2 tablespoons Spread Yourself Thin (page 141),
¾ cup broccoli or carrots

Dinner

The Weight-Loss Burger (page 138)

Snack #3

Yogi Pops (page 141)

SUNDAY: 1,150 CALORIES PLUS CHEAT MEAL

Breakfast

The 'Bama Bowl (page 121), ½ cup orange juice

Snack #1

4 ounces Lemon Drips and Drops smoothie (page 116)

Lunch

Hurry Curry (page 125)

Snack

4 to 8 ounces Lemon Drips and Drops smoothie (page 116),
1 cup melon

Dinner

Cheat meal

Perfect Week, Sample 2

MONDAY: 1,457 CALORIES

Breakfast

One glass (8 ounces) Abs Diet Ultimate Power Smoothie
(page 113); make extra for later

Snack #1

1 teaspoon peanut butter, raw vegetables (as much as
you want)

Lunch

Turkey or roast beef sandwich on whole-grain bread,
1 cup 1 percent or fat-free milk, 1 apple

Snack #2

1 ounce almonds, 1 ½ cups berries

Dinner

Italian Chowin' (page 129)

Snack #3

4 ounces Abs Diet Ultimate Power Smoothie

TUESDAY: 1,450 CALORIES

Breakfast

Eggs Beneficial Sandwich (page 118), 1 cup fat-free milk

Snack #1

1 teaspoon peanut butter, 1 bowl oatmeal or high-fiber cereal

Lunch

The I-Am-Not-Eating-Salad Salad (page 122)

Snack #2

3 slices deli turkey, 1 large orange

Dinner

Brazilian Chicken (page 130)

Snack #3

1 ounce almonds, 4 ounces cantaloupe

WEDNESDAY: 1,390 CALORIES

Breakfast

One glass (8 ounces) Halle Berries smoothie (page 113); make extra for later

Snack #1

1 ounce raisins

Lunch

Guac and Roll (page 123)

Snack #2

1 stick string cheese, raw vegetables (as much as you want)

Dinner

Salmon Rushdie (page 132)

Snack #3

4 to 8 ounces Halle Berries smoothie

THURSDAY: 1,480 CALORIES

Breakfast

1 slice whole-grain bread with 1 teaspoon peanut butter, ½ cup All-Bran cereal with 1 cup 1 percent or fat-free milk, 1 cup berries

Snack #1

8 ounces low-fat yogurt, 1 can low-sodium V8 juice

Lunch

Guilt-Free BLT (page 123)

Snack #2

3 slices lean deli roast beef, 1 large orange

Dinner

Terra Ricotta (page 135)

Snack #3

1 teaspoon peanut butter, ½ cup low-fat ice cream

FRIDAY: 1,660 CALORIES

Breakfast

One glass (8 ounces) Banana Split smoothie (page 113); make extra for later

Snack #1

1 ounce almonds, 4 ounces cantaloupe

Lunch

Hot Tuna (page 124)

Snack #2

3 slices lean deli roast beef, 1 large orange

Dinner

Chili Con Turkey (page 131)

Snack #3

4 ounces Banana Split smoothie

SATURDAY: 1,090 CALORIES PLUS CHEAT MEAL

Breakfast

One glass (8 ounces) Halle Berries smoothie (page 113); make extra for later

Snack #1

1 cup high-fiber cereal, 1 cup low-fat yogurt

Lunch

Leftover Chili Con Turkey

Snack #2

1 teaspoon peanut butter, 1 or 2 slices whole-grain bread

Dinner

Cheat meal! Have whatever you've been craving this week: wine and cheese, burgers, fillet of whatever—anything you can dream of.

||||||||||||||||||||||||||||||||||||||||||||||||||||||||||||||||||||||||||||||||||||||||||||||||||||||||||||||

6 Surprising Foods With Health Benefits

1. Iceberg Lettuce. Did you think it was a nutritional weakling? Most people do, yet it turns out that half a head contains significantly more alpha-carotene, a powerful disease-fighting antioxidant, than either romaine lettuce or spinach.

2. Pork Chops. Purdue University researchers found that a 6-ounce serving daily of the other white meat helped people preserve their muscle while losing weight.

3. Mushrooms. When you digest mushrooms, metabolites are created that have been shown to boost immunity and prevent cancer growth, according to researchers in the Netherlands.

4. Red-Pepper Flakes. A Dutch study shows that by consuming about half a teaspoon of red pepper 30 minutes prior to a meal, you can reduce calorie intake by 16 percent. Plus, new research shows that the active ingredient capsaicin in hot peppers may help kill cancer cells.

5. Full-Fat Cheese. You know that dairy is one of the 12 Abs Diet Powerfoods, but full-fat cheese? Yes. It's an excellent source of casein protein, one of the best muscle-building nutrients you can eat.

6. Vinegar. Sprinkle it on your sandwich. Scientists in Sweden discovered that when people ate 2 tablespoons of vinegar with a meal high in carbohydrates, their blood sugar was 23 percent lower than when they skipped the antioxidant-loaded liquid.

Snack #3

4 ounces Halle Berries smoothie

SUNDAY: 1,530 CALORIES

Breakfast

The I-Haven't-Had-My-Coffee-Yet Sandwich (page 119)

Snack #1

1 teaspoon peanut butter, 1 can low-sodium V8 juice

Brunch (relax—it's Sunday):

2 scrambled eggs, 2 slices whole-grain toast,
1 banana, 1 cup 1 percent or fat-free milk

Snack #2

2 slices lean deli roast beef, 1 slice fat-free cheese

Dinner

BBQ King (page 132)

Snack #3

1 ounce almonds, ½ cup low-fat ice cream

Perfect Week, Sample 3

MONDAY: 1,592 CALORIES

Breakfast

3-egg-white omelet with chopped vegetables,
1 whole-wheat English muffin with 2 teaspoons
soft margarine

Snack #1

Raw mixed vegetables, ¼ cup hummus

Lunch

3 ounces sliced turkey breast in a whole-wheat tortilla
with mixed greens, tomato, and 2 or 3 slices of
avocado; 1 cup mixed green salad with 2 teaspoons
olive oil and vinegar

Snack #2

1 cup berries mixed with 2 tablespoons fat-free plain yogurt

Dinner

Asian chicken salad: 2 cups mixed greens, red onions, and tomato wedges; 3 ounces cooked chicken breast, sliced; ½ cup mandarin orange sections; and 1 ounce cashews tossed with 1 tablespoon olive oil and vinegar; 4 whole-grain crackers

Snack #3

1 piece fruit, 1 cup fat-free plain or artificially sweetened yogurt

TUESDAY: 1,597 CALORIES

Breakfast

1 cup whole-grain cereal with 2 tablespoons raisins and 1 cup fat-free or 1 percent milk, 1 banana

Snack #1

1 container fat-free plain yogurt mixed with 2 tablespoons dried fruit and 2 teaspoons honey

Lunch

1 cup broth-based or tomato soup; 2 ounces sliced lean roast beef with lettuce, tomato, and mustard on 2 slices of whole-wheat bread

Snack #2

1 stick string cheese, 2 whole-wheat crackers

Dinner

1 cup cooked white or brown rice, 3 ounces grilled shrimp in gumbo sauce, mixed green salad with 2 teaspoons olive oil and vinegar

Snack #3

1 large whole-wheat pretzel

WEDNESDAY: 1,427 CALORIES

Breakfast

1 cup oatmeal with 2 tablespoons mixed dried fruit and nuts and 1 teaspoon cinnamon, ¼ cup fat-free plain yogurt, 1 cup orange or grapefruit juice

Snack #1

¼ cup microwave air-popped popcorn (100 calories' worth; see package)

Lunch

tuna salad: 3 ounces grilled or canned tuna, 5 small red potatoes, ½ cup string beans, and 5 to 8 olives on a bed of salad greens tossed with 2 teaspoons olive oil and 1 tablespoon red-wine vinegar

Snack #2

1 large rectangular graham cracker with 1 teaspoon nut butter, 1 piece fruit

Dinner

1 vegetarian burger with lettuce, tomato, and red onion on a soft wheat roll; side salad of mixed greens and vegetables and 2 teaspoons olive oil and vinegar dressing

Snack #3

½ cup fat-free ice cream or frozen yogurt

THURSDAY: 1,564 CALORIES

Breakfast

¾ cup muesli with 1 cup fat-free milk, 1 orange or ½ grapefruit

Snack #1

1 ounce low-fat cheese, 2 whole-wheat crackers

Lunch

tossed salad: mixed salad greens, cucumber, red bell pepper, red onion, diced carrots, tomato, ½ cup chickpeas, ½ cup string beans, and 1 ounce grated hard cheese tossed with 2 teaspoons olive oil and 1 tablespoon red-wine vinegar; 1 small whole-wheat roll

Snack #2

1 cup fortified soy milk, 2 Whole Grain Fig Newton cookies

Dinner

spaghetti marinara: 1 cup cooked whole-grain pasta topped with ½ cup marinara sauce and 1 tablespoon grated Romano cheese, side salad with olive oil and vinegar or light dressing

Snack #3

2 kiwifruits

FRIDAY: 1,115 CALORIES PLUS CHEAT MEAL

Breakfast

1 cup hot oatmeal with ¼ cup fat-free plain yogurt and 2 tablespoons raisins

Snack #1

1 energy bar like a PowerBar Pria or a Luna bar

Lunch

2 ounces whole-wheat pita, 2 ounces chicken or turkey breast, 1 tablespoon cranberry sauce with chopped mixed greens

Snack #2

1 container fat-free fruit-flavored yogurt with banana

Dinner

Cheat meal

Snack #3

1 low-fat or fat-free brownie, 1 cup fat-free milk

SATURDAY: 1,557 CALORIES

Breakfast

2 eggs and 1 egg white, scrambled; 2 slices whole-wheat toast with 2 teaspoons soft margarine and 1 tablespoon jam; ½ cup mixed fruit and ½ cup fat-free yogurt

Snack #1

½ whole-wheat pita with 1 tablespoon hummus

Lunch

1 cup chicken noodle soup, 4 whole-wheat crackers, mixed green salad with 1 tablespoon grated hard cheese and 5 sliced olives tossed with 2 teaspoons olive oil and vinegar

Snack #2

1½ cups watermelon chunks

Dinner

4 ounces broiled lean steak, ½ cup mashed potatoes (made with soft margarine), 1 cup steamed broccoli with 2 teaspoons Parmesan cheese

Snack #3

1 piece fresh fruit with ½ cup sorbet

SUNDAY: 1,448 CALORIES

Breakfast

2 whole-wheat frozen toaster waffles topped with 1 tablespoon nut butter and ½ medium banana, sliced; 1 cup fat-free milk

Snack #1

8 ounces low-fat yogurt

Lunch

1 medium baked potato topped with sautéed mixed vegetables (e.g., mushrooms, onions, broccoli) in 1 tablespoon olive oil with 1 ounce grated hard cheese

Snack #2

10 almonds or cashews

Dinner

turkey or chicken burger: 4 ounces grilled or broiled chicken or turkey (white meat only) with onions, tomatoes, and lettuce on whole-wheat roll; mixed greens tossed with 2 teaspoons olive oil and vinegar

Snack #3

1 4-ounce fat-free pudding

Chapter 11

ABS DIET ADAPTATIONS

Tailoring the Plan for Each Woman's
Individual Needs

THE ROADBLOCK TO ANY
successful weight-loss plan is clearly marked with a capital I: Inconvenience.
If a diet doesn't fit into your work hours, your lifestyle, your health, or your
habits, then it's going to fail faster than a Rob Schneider movie. Going to Subway for virtually every meal isn't convenient for most people, nor is cooking
up a pound of bacon every morning for breakfast, nor is asking the server at a
restaurant to pop a frozen dinner into the microwave and nuke it for 3 minutes.
A lot of diets simply aren't that convenient to follow. I believe that the Abs Diet
is convenient—because it gives you enough guidelines to help you understand
what healthy eating is while also giving you enough flexibility to make it work
for you whether you eat at home, out, in the car, or while watching your kids'
soccer and ballet practices.

That said, sticking to a diet—or, rather, changing your eating lifestyle—isn't
just a matter of how it fits into your schedule but also how it fits into your life and
into your body. Women's needs may be a little different than those of the typical
guy—namely, you're likely a little more tuned in to your health than he is, and
there are certain biological fundamentals that make your body different than

his (more on hormones and pregnancy in later chapters). And that's why I want to outline some strategies that may be of help to women in particular—based on feedback I've heard from women about what they want in addition to the fundamental principles, strategies, and recipes of the Abs Diet.

So, here, I'd like to outline some of the things you can do to make the six major Abs Diet principles work to complement your life, your personality, and your health—and not compete against them.

If You're a Calorie Counter . . .

PERSONALLY, I'D RATHER watch aforementioned Rob Schneider movies than count calories—too tedious a job and too inexact a science if you're eating on the run. But I also realize that many of you like to count calories for a couple of reasons: Mainly, doing so can really help give you a fairly accurate gauge of whether you're staying in your optimum caloric range (especially because your caloric requirements are lower than men's and because all of us tend to miscalculate portion sizes). In the major Abs Diet guidelines I laid out in Chapter 7, I explained that eating powerfoods is really one way to let the foods count calories for you—if you eat a balance of good, healthy foods six times a day. That doesn't mean that you can't count calories if that works best with your personality. So if you're going to be a calorie counter, you need to arm yourself with three tools to help make counting as manageable as possible.

1. **A food diary.** Write down everything you eat and drink as you consume it. The only way to accurately tally is to keep a running list, rather than trying to remember at the end of the day.

2. **Measuring cups and food scales.** The fact is, most of us underestimate the amount of food we actually eat (thanks, in large part, to restaurants that serve about 133 serving sizes in one dinner entrée). After a few weeks of measuring out cereal and weighing your fish, you'll be much better at eyeballing and dividing up accurate serving and portion sizes.

3. **A comprehensive listing of calories,** so you can quickly find what you need. Luckily, this one's easy. Yours begins on page 362.

Some other things to think about if you're going to include calorie tallying as part of the Abs Diet:

Estimate your caloric needs. As evidenced by cars and super-models, not everything is built in the same way. To figure out how many calories you need to maintain your current weight, multiply your weight in pounds by 11 and add 200 to 300 if you exercise regularly. For example, a sedentary 155-pound woman needs about 1,705 calories a day; an active one might need 2,005. (For

||||||||||||||||||||||||||||||||||||||||||||||||||||||||||||||||||||||||||||||||||||||||||||

What's a 100-Calorie Portion?

Proteins

2 ounces or 2 slices low-fat American or Cheddar cheese

2 slices bacon

2 ounces chicken (no skin)

2 small eggs

1½ cups fat-free milk

1 cup 1 percent milk

½ ounce roasted peanuts

2 ounces pork

2 ounces salmon or tuna

4 ounces (about 15) shrimp

Fats

1 tablespoon butter

2 teaspoons olive or corn oil

1 tablespoon mayo

1 tablespoon peanut butter

Carbs

¾ cup All-Bran cereal

1 large apple

1 medium banana

2 cups (about 50) green beans

½ cup corn

¾ cup plain oatmeal

1 ounce pasta

½ medium baked potato

20 medium strawberries

8 teaspoons sugar

2½ slices low-calorie wheat bread

a more detailed formula that's tailored to your body, flip back to page 69.) Then decide how fast you want to lose the weight. A pound of body weight equals 3,500 calories, so you would need to shave 500 a day from your count to drop a pound a week. The best balance, according to a review of studies on diet composition in the *Journal of the American Dietetic Association,* is 35 to 50 percent carbs, 25 to 35 percent fat, and about 25 to 30 percent protein.

Fiber up. If you're making every calorie count, your best play is to make sure you're going heavy on the high-fiber foods. That's because foods rich in water and fiber are bulkier but less caloric. A cup of strawberries, for example, has about the same calorie content as a small cookie but is far more satisfying. In one study at Pennsylvania State University, women ate the same weight of food over a 2-day period. When the women ate higher-fiber foods on the second day, they took in 30 percent fewer calories but didn't feel any hungrier or less full.

Stick to the six. A British study found that women who ate the same number of meals every day ate fewer calories than those who changed it up from day to day and sometimes skipped breakfast or worked through lunch or ate dessert and then a late-night snack. Plus, when the women ate inconsistently, their metabolisms slowed.

Get to know your servings. Most portion sizes from restaurants and take-out places are well beyond an acceptable serving size. You need to start thinking that those dishes are two (or three) meals instead of one. Review the Abs Diet Portion-Distortion Decoder on page 2. Also, when you cook meals, serve them up on small plates: Less food will look like more, and you'll eat less.

Don't fear the frozens. Not all frozen foods are the nutritional equivalent of the boxes they come in. Some are healthy (find ones with low trans fats, saturated fats, sugars, and high-fructose corn syrup). The best part is that they enforce a calorie ceiling on you. A study in the *International Journal of Obesity* showed that people who regularly use meal replacements such as Slim-Fast and Healthy Choice lose nearly twice as much weight as those on a low-calorie diet. Why? Because those meals have preset portions and a controlled number of calories.

Know the most satisfying foods. In what seems to be a bit of voodoo math, 1 calorie doesn't always equal one calorie—because of the effect that foods have on how much you want to eat later. Australian researchers developed a satiety index to determine how satisfied you feel after eating. Study participants ate a 240-calorie portion of each food, then rated their satiety over 2 hours. These are the most satisfying foods (notice how many power-foods made the list!), so they help you control hunger and decrease your calories during the day.

White potatoes	Fish	Beef
Eggs	Soup	Salad
Oatmeal	Apples	Popcorn
Beans		

If You're a Vegetarian . . .

BEING A VEGETARIAN has a lot of benefits besides never having to endure the 2-hour wait for a table at the popular steak joint. Not only do vegetarians who eat dairy products and eggs typically get their essential vitamins and minerals but—not surprisingly—research also finds that vegetarians typically eat more nutrient-rich fruits, vegetables, legumes, nuts, and whole grains than meat-eaters do. They also tend to eat less fat, including unhealthy saturated fat, and are less likely to be overweight. Because many of the Abs Diet Powerfoods are vegetarian-friendly, you can follow the same principles I've outlined, so long as you keep in mind some special considerations.

Get enough protein. Because you won't be getting your all-important protein in the form of lean meats, make sure you get at least three daily servings of protein-packed, low-fat dairy products such as milk and yogurt (in addition to cheese), as well as two to three eggs per week. When scientists from McMaster University in Ontario assessed the food intake of 617 dieters, they found that eating more protein can reduce the amount of fat around your midsection. Specifically, people who consumed an average of 20 grams of extra protein per day lowered their waist-to-hip ratio measurements by 24 percent, compared with dieters who ate more carbs.

Go nuts. Nuts are also good sources of protein, healthy fats, vitamins, and minerals. Walnuts, canola oil, and flaxseed can replace fish because they are good sources of heart-healthy omega-3 fatty acids.

Savor the soy. The good part about skipping meat is that you're also skipping the cuts that have more blubber than a Sea World tank. The FDA recommends getting at least 25 grams of soy protein each day (for its cardiovascular and other health benefits). It's easy to get, too: 8 ounces of soy milk contains 8 grams of soy protein, one soy burger contains 10 grams, and ¼ cup of soy nuts contains 12 grams. Another option: Green vegetable soybeans (edamame) make a healthy, satisfying snack.

Take your vitamins. A German study found levels of vitamin B12 low enough to cause attention, mood, and thinking problems in 68 percent of vegetarians and low enough to raise blood homocysteine (a risk factor for heart disease, dementia, and Alzheimer's) in 38 percent. Remedy: a daily multivitamin with 100 percent of the daily value for B12 (6 micrograms).

Pump some dietary iron. Only 2 to 10 percent of the iron in plants is absorbed by your digestive tract, so drink a glass of high-vitamin C juice (citrus or tomato) at the same meal as high-iron foods such as beans, because vitamin C can unlock iron from plants.

Remember, you don't have license to gorge. Just because you're not eating fatty cuts of meat doesn't mean you can make an all-out food fest of chips, bread, baked goods, cookies, crackers, and sweets that are allowed on vegetarian diets.

If You're Lactose Intolerant . . .

IF YOUR BODY can't digest the sugar that's in milk, it's likely that those darn milk mustaches aren't the only things that disturb you. You're probably looking at the dairy products (and their amazing benefits) on the list of powerfoods and wondering if there's another way you can get those same benefits.

It's true that people who are lactose intolerant don't typically get enough calcium (about 700 milligrams a day, compared with the 1,200 that are recommended for healthy bones). And that can be a problem: Besides the bone-building benefits of calcium, you also want it for the effects it seems to have on weight loss. If dairy leaves you gassy, crampy, and bloated, you can avoid a calcium deficit in these ways.

▶ Drink milk made for people with lactose intolerance, such as Lactaid.

▶ Try yogurt; the enzymes it contains digest milk sugar for you.

▶ Take a calcium supplement, plus 400 IU of vitamin D.

▶ Eat nondairy foods that have lots of calcium, such as sardines, almonds, and broccoli.

▶ Snack on Cheddar or Swiss cheese—two naturally low-lactose cheeses.

If You've Got IBS . . .

I KNOW IT sounds like a government agency or a new TV station, but IBS (irritable bowel syndrome) is something that disturbs 50 million Americans—about 75 percent of whom are women, according to the US Department of Health and Human Services. In normal digestion, the walls of your intestines contract and then relax as they transport food from your stomach. When you have IBS, the contractions are stronger and longer, causing diarrhea, constipation, or bouts of both. It's not clear why women are so disproportionately affected by the condition, but researchers suspect it may be related to hormone fluctuations throughout the menstrual cycle. In any case, here's what you can do to help with the pain.

▶ Eating your six smaller meals a day will help naturally by keeping you from overloading your digestive tract with larger amounts of food three times a day.

▶ Limit your consumption of fructose, a sugar found in fruits and most refined foods. Research shows that fructose is related to more severe symptoms of IBS.

▶ Keep a journal to track which foods cause the most discomfort. Researchers at St. George's Hospital in London analyzed blood samples from 108 IBS patients and 43 healthy folks to check their reactions to 16 foods, including nuts, meat, dairy, and grains. More severe reactions were triggered by wheat, beef, pork, and lamb. Surprisingly, dairy products—a group anecdotally linked to IBS—caused no problems. If you have IBS, cut back on meat and wheat, and keep a diary to pinpoint which foods cause distress.

▶ The herb peppermint relaxes the digestive tract's smooth muscles, easing spasms. German research found that capsules containing 180 to 200 milligrams of peppermint oil eased IBS pain, bloating, and gas for 58 percent of takers. Look for capsules with an enteric coating that helps prevent them from causing heartburn. Take one with a glass of water before dinner.

▶ Make sure to stick to your workouts. Physical activity helps regulate those intestinal contractions. A University of Washington study found that those people with IBS who exercised regularly had fewer symptoms than those who didn't.

If You're On Antidepressants...

THESE DAYS, ANTIDEPRESSANTS seem almost as prevalent as iPods. Doctors prescribe them for a number of reasons, including depression, libido issues,

||||||||||||||||||||||||||||||||||||||||||||||||||||||||||||||||||||||||||||||||||||||||||||||||||||||||||||

Lose Weight in Your Sleep

A 2009 study in the *American Journal of Public Health* found that people who get enough sleep to feel rested have healthier diets than those who get insufficient sleep. The researchers say sleep-deprived people exhibit lower levels of leptin (the hormone that suppresses appetite) and higher levels of ghrelin (the hormone that makes you hungry). Try these sleep strategies.

▶ Aim for 7 or more hours of sleep each night. A large study of adults found that people who sleep at least 7 hours have the lowest risk of mortality.

▶ Exercise in the afternoon. It can take 6 hours for your body temperature to cool enough to promote sleep onset after exercising.

▶ Avoid caffeine within 8 hours of bedtime and eating within 2. The National Sleep Foundation says both stimulate your system, making it difficult to both get to sleep and control your weight.

and smoking cessation. While some antidepressants are weight neutral, others (such as classes of drugs called SSRIs) can actually make you gain weight. Talk to your doctor about getting a new drug with the same antidepressant effect but without the weight gain. One medication that seems to even have a weight-loss effect is Bupropion. In a study of 422 overweight people, those taking Bupropion lost nearly 10 pounds, while those on a placebo lost about 3½ pounds.

If You're Likely to Give In to Temptation . . .

HOWEVER YOU SPEND your days—whether you work out of the house, whether you work in the house, whether you're running a business, or whether you're running a household—I have no doubt that you're multitasking. You're trying to get kids here and there, trying to advance your career, and reeling from all the technology that's supposed to make our lives easier. (How much chocolate did you down the last time your computer crashed?) The effect: We're under the gun. All the time. Sometimes, the only solace we can get from the rigors of life is in the refrigerator. And that, my friends, is clinically classified as Not Good. Here's how to deal with some of the stresses and temptations in life so that you don't make your waist pay the price for your stress.

Working late in the office: Keep fiber-rich snacks such as Country Choice's Oatmeal Squares or Luna bars in your desk drawer. Fiber, as opposed to an instant sugar rush, takes more time to release glucose into your bloodstream. This will keep you energized and full longer, plus improve brain function and productivity.

Feeding the kids: It may be tempting to snort up the last 10 fries or scoop out a few spoonfuls of SpaghettiOs, but they're just going to add on extra calories without nutrients. Anything your kid doesn't finish (and can't eat later) should immediately be thrown away so that you don't clean the plate. Also, buy snacks high in calcium, such as chocolate milk, low-fat yogurt, or string cheese, so that if you do pick from their plates, at least you're not doing so with Ding Dongs.

Partying with coworkers: Eat an apple and a handful of nuts an hour before you go so you won't feel like gorging on three-story appetizers when you get there.

If You're a Believer in the Theory That
Little Things Count . . .

IF YOU'RE WORKING with a daily calorie intake of somewhere in the neighborhood of 1,400 to 1,600 calories, then yes, every calorie does count. The following little tricks may not seem like they have a huge effect, but when you add up these changes over a period of time, they'll translate into a leaner and stronger body.

Sit down when eating. University of Minnesota researchers found that eating on the go caused women to consume more saturated fat and high calorie soft drinks than those who took the time to enjoy their meals sitting down.

Blot. Use a paper napkin to blot a teaspoon of fat off a pizza slice. At a slice a week, that's more than a whole cup of fat you won't eat—or wear—this year.

Tighten your belt. When you feel a craving and temptation to gorge, tighten your belt a notch—as a reminder of the size you'd like to be.

Get more milk. Consuming 1,800 milligrams of calcium a day could block the absorption of about 80 calories. Fill your coffee mug with skim or 1 percent milk, drink it down to the level you want in your coffee, then pour in your caffeine fix.

Buy cut veggies. They cost more, but they'll pay dividends later—because you're more likely to snack on them than on some other, less healthy food.

Get water down. A German study showed that drinking water burns calories. Drinking about 2 cups of cold water—no warmer than 72 degrees—used up roughly 25 calories. Drink a liter a day and you're talking 5 pounds a year.

Dilute juice. Add water to your fruit juice to reduce calories.

Make your drinks count. Have a V8 or tomato juice instead of a Diet Coke.

Have a power snack prepared. Mix three different kinds of beans and sprinkle in some low-cal Italian dressing. Have it as a snack all week.

Think about eating. Eat without doing anything else—no TV, no reading, no working.

Stop mindless snacking. Chew a strong-flavored gum like cinnamon while you're cooking. Sneaking a taste of the food will be less appealing.

|||||||||||||||||||||||||||||||||||||||||||||||||||||||||||||||||||||||||||||||||||||||||||||||||||||||||||||||

Your Perfect Vitamin

Though not every multivitamin/mineral will meet all your nutritional needs, yours should include these nutrients. Clip this list to see how your multi stacks up, or take it with you if you're shopping for a new multi.

NUTRIENT	AMOUNT PER TABLET
Vitamin A	5,000 IU
Beta-carotene	20 percent of vitamin A
Vitamin D	200 IU
Vitamin E	30 IU
Vitamin K	90 mcg
Folic acid	400 mcg
Vitamin B6	2 mg
Vitamin B12	2.4 mcg
Vitamin C	75 mg
Calcium	1,000 mg
Chromium	25 mcg
Copper	2 mg
Iron	18 mg
Magnesium	400 mg
Omega-3 fats	1 g
Selenium	55 mcg
Zinc	8 mg

Special Bonus Section

WHAT'S ON YOUR MIND?

Psychological Strategies for Dealing with Your
Obstacles—And Your Changing Moods

T HERE'S A REASON WHY
there are more diet plans than there are American Idol wannabes: because
many of them are pretty darn lousy. Why? Not necessarily because of the food
plan and nutritional choices (though there are plenty of those that are lousy),
but many times because of all the other stuff that comes with the nutritional
nuts and bolts. That is, how does what's happening in your mind affect what's
happening in your stomach? How realistic is it to think that you can stick to
the diet over the long term? How low maintenance is the actual plan?

I believe that the Abs Diet goes a long way toward eliminating some of the
intangible issues that often come with dieting. For example, the once-a-week
cheat meal allows you to give in to temptations so you're not constantly denying
yourself a hunk of 32-cheese lasagna. The six meals a day keep you from feeling starved and frustrated. And the delicious smoothies satisfy the daily cravings for sweets—a satisfaction that's absent from so many diet plans. That said,
I know that anytime you make a change in your approach to eating or exercise,
you're going to face more obstacles than a boot-camp recruit. And I believe that

much of your success will come not only from following the guidelines and principles of the Abs Diet but also from having some strategies to cope with the psychological aspects of changing the way you eat and the way you exercise.

Struggle 1: Feeling Full Versus Feeling Starving

WE'VE BEEN CONDITIONED to believe that the only way we're supposed to feel on a diet is starving, famished, and about 3 seconds away from gnawing on the drywall. Somehow, denying ourselves food makes us feel like we're accomplishing something. But the fact is, the more you starve yourself, the more you slow your metabolism, and the more weight you're going to end up gaining.

On the flip side, you don't want to live your whole life feeling like you just finished Thanksgiving dinner. You shouldn't feel bloated, gross, and ready to pop. The feeling you want is somewhere in the middle—in a state of nutritional satisfaction.

When following the Abs Diet dictum of eating six times a day, that satisfaction is what you should feel. But it may take some time for you to make the adjustment—because you're not used to feeling satisfied when you're "on a diet."

One of the best ways to reset your satiety clock is to make sure you don't skimp on breakfast. Researchers in the Netherlands found that those who started the day with a high-calorie meal rich in complex carbohydrates were more likely to feel satisfied for longer. Aim for a breakfast that's 20 percent of your caloric needs for the day (about 350 calories) and full of slow-burning complex carbs. That means a bowl of raisin bran and one slice of whole-wheat toast with all-fruit preserves, or a half cup of multigrain oatmeal and half a sliced banana sprinkled into a small container of low-fat vanilla yogurt. It may take a few weeks to retrain your mind into thinking that staying in a state of satisfaction is good for you. But if you can set your stomach up for a perfect day of eating, you'll have a better shot of doing the same for your mind.

Struggle 2: You're Edgy When
You're Just Starting Out

IT'S NO SECRET that going on a diet can be as tough on your mind as it is on your local ice-cream shop: A recent UCLA study linked dieting to chronic stress. Not only can it make you revert to your old eating habits but it can also keep you fat because cortisol, a hormone released during stress, slows down weight loss. This is when you need to rely on your friends for support—or even ask them to join you in your weight-loss crusade. Researchers from the United Kingdom found that women who dieted as part of a group had less stress than those who went it alone.

The good news is that the uncomfortable feeling you experience when you first adjust your eating routine should last only a little while; it takes only 21 days for a repeated action to become a natural habit.

Struggle 3: Your PMS Munchies Have You Craving Cheat Meals More Than Once a Week

DURING THE FINAL 14 days of your menstrual cycle, progesterone is elevated. When that happens, the feel-good hormone serotonin decreases, along with endorphins and dopamine, two chemicals responsible for helping your body fight stress. The combination makes your mood plummet and your appetite soar. This is why it's especially important to stick to your six meals. Eating often helps stabilize your blood sugar, cut fatigue, and prevent bloating. You'll find more on combating PMS and other hormone-related eating habits in Chapter 16.

|||||||||||||||||||||||||||||||||||||||||||||||||||||||||||||||||||||||||||||||||||||||||||||||||||||||||||||||||

Workout Struggles

We all have times when it's tough to psych ourselves up for our workout routines. Here's a rundown of the most common workout obstacles and the best ways to get past them.

Strength training: So what if it's 8 reps or 12? Whether you're doing crunches, bench presses, or lunges, it's easy to lose motivation when you're doing rep after rep after rep.

The Fix: Keep your eye on your goals. You build strength when your muscles break down and your body repairs them by creating tougher muscle tissue. You barely begin to break down muscles during the first few reps, which is why you need to pick a weight that allows you to complete 10 challenging yet doable reps without compromising form.

Running: Sore legs. If your body is producing lactic acid during one of the interval sessions that you'll learn about on page 212, it can cause a burning sensation in your

Struggle 4: You're Not Seeing the Scale Move

AFTER ABOUT 6 weeks of steady exercise, you'll notice that you have more muscle and less fat—even if the number on the scale hasn't changed. That's because muscle weighs more than fat. So you have to remember that even though your weight might not be dropping, you're still making progress. Your new muscle is helping you burn even more fat because, as you remember, muscle tissue uses more calories than fat cells do. So the more muscle you possess, the more calories you'll burn—even when you're not working out.

Look at other ways to measure your progress besides your scale, such as the way your clothes fit, or an improvement in the amount of exercise you do, or changes in the size of your body parts. Save the scale for once-a-month measurements if you're easily frustrated by small changes in weight.

Your Mood, Your Meal

THERE ARE A lot of things that can change your mood for the better—a beautiful sunset, a productive workout, a flirty e-mail sent at the right time by the right person. There are also a lot of things that can do the opposite—a gray sky, a twisted ankle, or a snarky e-mail sent at the wrong time by the wrong

||||||||||||||||||||||||||||||||||||||||||||||||||||||||||||||||||||||||||||||||||||||||||||||||||||||||||

quads and glutes. That soreness is pain you can push through and a positive indicator of how hard you're working.

The Fix: Resting for a minute or two will allow your body to take in more oxygen, which you need to help flush the lactic acid. Stretch while you rest to separate the muscle fibers and improve circulation. Try the Stork to stretch quads and hips: Stand on one leg and pull the other behind you, bringing your heel toward your butt.

Cardio machines: Boring! Your brain is zoning out, and your body needs new stimulation as it adapts to repetitive movement patterns.

The Fix: All the more reason to make sure your cardio workouts are interval sessions. They'll trick your mind into thinking the workout is moving quicker, and you'll challenge your muscles, burning more calories and building strength. Do 2 minutes at a fast pace, then drop it down for 1 minute, alternating until you're suddenly out of time.

person. It's no secret that our moods can swing faster than a 7-year-old at a playground, but one of the tricks for battling out of a bad mood or foul feelings is using nature's medicine—food—to your advantage. By eating the healthy foods that can pick you up, you help your mind—without hurting your body.

When you're blue: The thing you may reach for when you're feeling a little on the weepy side may be the hunk of stashed chocolate (left cupboard, third shelf, am I right?). That may give you an immediate sugar jolt, but you should choose something with a little more of a lasting effect. Go for a low-fat, low-protein, high-carbohydrate snack: Think toasted whole-wheat English muffin with a dollop of blueberry all-fruit preserves (or better, fresh blueberries). When high-carb foods aren't bogged down by protein or fat, they allow that amino acid called tryptophan (you know it from turkey) to flood into your brain, where it morphs into serotonin, a neurotransmitter that boosts mood and curbs food cravings. A bowl of air-popped popcorn is another good alternative.

When you're depressed: It's all about the fish. More and more evidence says that omega-3 fatty acids may help ease symptoms associated with depression. Omega-3s are found in fatty fish such as salmon, herring, and tuna. One study, for example, showed that eating fish twice a week was associated with a lower risk of depression. If you're concerned about mercury (which is relatively high in fatty fish), stick to wild Pacific salmon, shrimp, summer flounder, farmed catfish, croaker, haddock, and mid-Atlantic blue crab, all of which contain omega-3s but are low in mercury.

When you're feeling dull: Here's the perfect place for your cup of joe (minus the whipped cream and flavors that sound like they belong in a bakery). Within a half hour of drinking a cup, your nervous system gets revved and you feel alert and better able to concentrate. How? The caffeine short-circuits a nerve chemical called adenosine that blocks your energy-boosting brain chemicals, helping you get a healthy rush. Just don't get into the cycle where you need coffee to pick you up, then feel a letdown, then reach for more coffee, and so on. To maintain a pleasant, temporary buzz, limit yourself to no more than three 5-ounce cups of coffee a day.

When you're sleepy: There's no doubt that a decrease in sleep equals an increase in irritability. To combat daytime fatigue, cut back on dinner. A big meal can keep you awake at night while your stomach churns on overload. Keep your dinner under 500 calories, and try to incorporate more foods containing the mineral copper. (Examples are chicken, bananas, and avocados.) There's some evidence that people who have a lower copper intake have a hard time getting to sleep and feel less rested when they wake up. Also add in a small low-fat, low-protein, high-carb evening snack (like a bit of sorbet or a small piece of fruit and graham crackers) to tap into serotonin's soothing effects.

When you're beyond tired: First off, if you're feeling too tired to even do your normal daily activities, you should see a doctor because fatigue can be a sign of a serious illness. It's one of the first signs of iron deficiency and anemia, the most common nutritional deficiency in the world, especially among women of childbearing age. The cause? Not getting enough iron from your food. As good as beans, grains, and vegetables are for you, the form of iron they provide is weak and hard to absorb. Animal protein not only contains more iron but also provides a special form that your body absorbs better than it does the iron from plants. If you're feeling listless, especially if you've cut back on meat, try eating shrimp, lean beef, dark chicken or turkey meat (without the skin), or fish. Adding a multivitamin with iron will also help. Another tactic: Try drinking more water. Chronic low fluid intake is a common but often overlooked cause of mild dehydration and fatigue.

Chapter 12

FITTING THE ABS DIET INTO EVERYDAY LIFE

How This Simple Eating Plan Makes Your Life Simpler, Too

I N PREVIOUS CHAPTERS, I
outlined why the Abs Diet for Women works—and will work for you, for life.
I gave an overview of the science and fed you some nifty terms like "glycemic
index" and "basal metabolism." And I listed a whole eating plan complete with
meals, snacks, and simple recipes.

But I also explained why most other diet plans are the nutritional equivalent of that tape recorder in *Mission: Impossible*—programmed to self-destruct
in 5 seconds or 5 weeks or 5 years. Most diets just aren't designed to last over
the long haul, or they're so complicated and restrictive that you'd have to quit
your day job and disown half your friends in order to follow them to the letter.
Many diets fail because they require us to work too hard and ignore the fact
that we're already working too hard. What most of us feel, every day, is that
our worlds are on the verge of spinning out of control. And what we want is to
take back control—of our lives, our careers, our relationships, our bodies, our
diets, ourselves.

One of the great side benefits of the Abs Diet is that it helps you reassert control over your life, which means taking control of your stress level. I can't emphasize strongly enough how important stress management is for your weight, your health, and the quality of life you'll lead.

That's because our bodies simply aren't designed to handle the stress of modern life. See, when stress hits, one of the first things your body does is jack up its production of adrenaline. Adrenaline causes fat cells all over your body to squirt their stores of fatty acids into your bloodstream to be used as energy. This was great back when stress meant a charging saber-toothed tiger or an attacking horde of barbarians and your fight-or-flight mechanism switched on. But it's not so great in today's society, where the only tigers and barbarians you have to handle are the ones who sign your paycheck or spit milk across the table. You don't flee or fight; you just bear down to handle the situation. Meanwhile, your adrenal glands are producing yet another hormone to handle all that freshly released fat. It's called cortisol, but I want you to call it by its nickname: the belly-fat hormone.

In one Yale study, researchers asked 42 overweight people to perform an hour of stressful tasks—math problems, puzzles, and speech making. All the while, their cortisol levels were measured. The subjects who carried their extra weight in their bellies were discovered to be secreting more cortisol while under pressure. The theory runs like this: Stress hits, adrenaline mobilizes

||||||||||||||||||||||||||||||||||||||||||||||||||||||||||||||||||||||||||||||||||||||||||||||||||||||

Sneaky Ways to Keep Restaurants from Sabotaging Your Diet

▶ Many chefs pour at least an ounce of butter (200 calories and 23 grams of fat) onto a steak just so the meat will look juicier. Ask in advance and tell the cook to lay off.

▶ Those harmless-looking shredded carrots that dress up your beef are probably deep-fried; 1/2 cup is 137 calories (four times that of raw carrots) and 12 grams of fat. Skip 'em.

▶ If you go to a restaurant that serves salads tossed with dressing, it's usually a much lighter coating than what most people end up dumping on themselves, even if you order it on the side.

fat from all over the body, and cortisol takes the unused portion and stashes it with extreme prejudice toward the abdominal region. In a study of 438 firefighters, the ones who said they worried about their financial security gained 11.2 pounds over 7 years, compared with an average of 7.4 pounds gained by nonworriers. The key to managing your midsection, then, is managing your stress. Here are a few proven ways to keep your head—and your abs—when people all around you are losing theirs.

Skip Letterman. A University of Chicago study published in the journal *Sleep* showed that people who slept only 4 hours had cortisol levels 37 percent higher than others who got a full 8 hours of shut-eye; those who stayed awake the whole night had levels 45 percent higher. Sleep specialists suggest that you strive for 8 hours per night.

Stop tossing and turning. How well you sleep matters, too. Another University of Chicago study showed that people who got plenty of deep sleep— the quality stuff without all the dreaming and rapid eye movement—secreted

---

ABS DIET SUCCESS STORY

"I'm on the Abs Diet for Life"

Name: Marian Nagel

Age: 44

Height: 5'6"

Starting weight: 148

6 weeks later: 136

As a mother of teenagers, Marian Nagel came to a point when she had to make a decision: "Do I want to be old and fat or old and healthy?"

So Nagel decided to get back in shape for herself—as well as to inspire her son to do so, too. After purchasing *Men's Health* to help him, Nagel learned about the Abs Diet, and they both tried it. She told her son, "This isn't a diet; it's a list of foods you need to eat more of." Within 6 weeks, Nagel's son dropped from 324 pounds to 292, and she dropped 12 pounds during the same time. (Since then, Nagel dropped down to 132, and she's now focused on losing just 4 more pounds.)

almost 65 percent more human growth hormone (HGH) than those who were short on good slumber. You want more HGH to help prevent the loss of muscle mass caused by cortisol.

Remember C, as in "crisis." If you're in a stressful time of life—wondering why the jury has been out so long, perhaps—load up on vitamin C. For managing stress, you probably top out the benefit with a daily intake of 1,000 milligrams, divided into small doses throughout the day.

Don't have that last drink. Booze dehydrates you. Your body thinks there's a water shortage emergency, which bumps up your cortisol. How much alcohol is too much? Most of the smart money says three drinks a day. Same dehydration idea applies to caffeine. For cortisol control, stick to 200 milligrams per day, about what you get in 2 cups of coffee.

Take the wheel. A sense of control over some of the stressors in your life helps. "If you blast a volunteer randomly with a noise, his stress hormones rise," says Robert Sapolsky, PhD, professor of biological and neurological

---

"Especially for women over 40, it gets harder and harder to lose that belly fat after having kids," says Nagel, who went from 27 percent body fat to about 20 during the initial part of the program and especially liked doing the interval training on a treadmill. "But I lost an incredible amount of inches. During the 6 weeks, I lost about 3½ inches off my waist. How nice it is to be curvy again. I see guys at the gym who can't do the abs work that I do."

Nagel also thinks the eating plan is perfect for women. "Women have a tendency to be nervous eaters more than men, and they assume they're going to eat more and take more calories if they eat six meals a day. But if you do it the proper way, you're nourishing your body, which speeds metabolism. You're eating to be sure your body is burning something all the time," Nagel says.

But for all the help the Abs Diet has given Nagel, she's especially happy for the way it's helped her son.

"The best thing for me is to set an example—not only to get myself in great shape but be a good example for him," Nagel says. "I absolutely love it, I'm still doing it; it's more of a lifestyle change than a temporary thing. I'm on the Abs Diet for life."

sciences at Stanford University. "But if you give him a button and tell him that pressing it will decrease the likelihood of the noise, there's a smaller stress response to the same sound." Getting organized, even in small ways, may help you feel more like the captain of your ship.

Make a plan. "People manage stress more effectively if they can believe that things are improving," says Sapolsky. So make sure you always have something you're looking forward to. Hope makes stress manageable.

Get spiritual. Remember the simple wisdom of Simone Weil: Any undivided attention is prayer. If we can stop the tumble in our heads and every day briefly commit our complete attention to something—a 10-foot putt, a 10-penny nail, or a 10-year-old child—we may acquire the serenity many find in formal faith.

Chapter 18 will give you other great strategies for achieving peace of mind.

Chapter 13

TURBOCHARGING THE NEW ABS DIET

How Exercise Can Strip Away Fat
and Add Lean Muscle

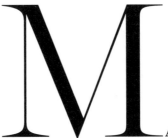AYBE THE PAST
few months, years, or decades of your life have been one big snowstorm—a snowstorm of office parties and happy hours, of vending machine dinners, of finishing the cake and ice cream off your children's plates. When you're a kid, those storms can be fun, but as you get older, they're more of a mess than anything else. They dump pounds and pounds of fat onto your thighs, hips, and once-flat stomach, leaving your abdominal muscles buried deep under everything. No sun's going to melt your fat after a couple of days, and no snowblower's going to suck it up and shoot it over to the neighbor's lawn. (But how cool would that be?)

If you want to see the sidewalk, you have to shovel the snow. If you want to find your abs and flatten your belly, you have to burn the fat.

Eating right is critical, and yes, by following the nutrition principles of the Abs Diet and centering your meals around the Abs Diet Powerfoods, you'll lose fat pretty effortlessly. But to maximize your weight loss and turn your fat into toned muscle, this book includes something other diet books ignore: a quick and easy exercise plan. Exercise will not only make you healthier; it'll also make you lose weight faster. It'll make you stronger. Most important, it'll make your body exchange your blobby fat for lean muscle—by converting energy that's stored in fat into energy that feeds muscle.

The New Abs Diet Workout Principles

HAVING WORKED AT *Men's Health* for more than 15 years, I know all the latest trends in exercise, but I also scour the latest and most credible scientific research measuring the effectiveness of various workout plans. With that knowledge, I've constructed the exercise portion of the plan to help you burn fat at the highest levels possible in the least amount of time. I know you don't have time to spend hours a day exercising, so I want you to get the most out of every workout. And I know that flexibility and convenience are the keys to formulating a plan you can stick to, so I've created a workout you can do at your local gym—or in your living room. This plan allows you to keep your workouts short and focused, while still keeping you on target for your ultimate goal. Pound for pound, it's the best workout possible for finding your abs and flattening your stomach. These are the workout principles.

|||||||||||||||||||||||||||||||||||||||||||||||||||||||||||||||||||||||||||||||||||||||||||||||||||||||

Quick Tips For Lean Abs

Move faster: Target your fast-twitch muscle fibers and you'll build stronger abs in less time. Spanish researchers found that doing abdominal exercises at a fast tempo activates more muscle than doing them slowly. Crank out as many reps as you can do in 20 seconds for a more effective core workout in less time.

Exercise, then eat: Research suggests that the best way to eat less at a meal is to work out right before it. This works in several ways: First, you're less hungry when your metabolism is revving, such as right after a workout. Second, you're thirstier, so you drink more water, which uses up space in your belly and relieves hunger. Third, the calories you do eat get burned for energy pronto—not stored as fat.

Stand taller: When you're walking, stand tall and picture a cape flowing off your shoulders, Superman-style, to ensure your best posture. A taller posture will give you the appearance of being slimmer, while also training your abs to stay firm.

Focus on your diet first. The first 2 weeks of exercise are optional. If you already exercise regularly, you can jump right into the Abs Diet Workout, and you should, because you'll burn even more fat than with the Abs Diet alone. But if you're a beginner or you haven't exercised in a long time, take the first 2 weeks to adjust to your new eating plan before starting the workout. If you're champing at the bit to begin maximizing your weight loss, start getting in the exercise habit by walking briskly for up to 30 minutes a day.

Focus on muscles. I know a lot of people who have tried to lose weight by running, but many of them don't accomplish that even after following a good running program. They've either stayed at the same weight or gained some. I think that happens for a couple of reasons. For one, steady-state cardiovascular exercise doesn't burn fat the way strength training does. Your muscles are hungry little suckers, and in order to keep themselves well nourished, they want to churn and burn those calories you're ingesting. So adding some muscle means you'll burn more calories—at the gym, on the job, even in bed. This program focuses on working your large muscle groups—your legs, chest, back, and shoulders—because that's where you can build the most muscle in the least amount of time (without adding a lot of bulk). Plus, when you work your larger muscles, you fire up your metabolism by creating a longer calorie afterburn—one that can last right up to your very next workout!

‖‖

Focus on the flip side: Your abs are an intricate system of muscles, connecting to your rib cage, your hips, and even your backbone. To have strong abs, you need not only belly exercises but also lower-back strength and exercises for your obliques (the abdominal muscles that run down the sides of your torso).

Practice looking leaner: Maybe you've heard of "muscle memory": the way your body learns to do a physical activity (like riding a bike) and never forgets. Well, your abs have a memory, too. If you consciously keep your abs firm throughout the day, they'll tend to stay firm even when you're relaxed.

Don't sacrifice your best ally: When you lose weight on a "diet," muscle is the first thing to go. It's more expensive for your body to retain than fat is, so when you run low on calories, your body dumps muscle mass and turns it into energy. (That's why diets of denial are counterproductive.) When you go off the diet, you begin to gain back the pounds—but because you now have less calorie-burning muscle, the weight you gain is fat. By dieting, you've effectively turned muscle into fat.

Think about the small fraction of time you spend exercising. Even if you work out four or five times a week for an hour at a time, that's nothing compared with the amount of time you're not exercising every day. So in order to gain the most metabolic benefit, you want to maximize the calories you're burning when you're not working out.

Focus on spending less time in the gym. The Abs Diet Workout employs two simple concepts to maximize muscle growth and fat-burning and minimize the time you spend exercising.

Circuit training. This term refers to the practice of performing different exercises one right after another. For example, we'll have you do a set of leg exercises followed immediately by a set of an upper-body exercise, until you do 8 to 10 different exercises in a row. There are two reasons circuit training works. First, by keeping you moving and cutting down the rest periods between exercises, circuit training keeps your heart rate elevated throughout your training session, maximizing your fat burn while providing tremendous

---

ABS DIET SUCCESS STORY

"The Proof Is in the Pants!"

Name: Jessica Guff

Age: 43

Height: 5'4"

Starting weight: 130

6 weeks later: 120

Jessica Guff doesn't believe in stepping on a scale. See, numbers don't give a total health picture, Guff says. What really matters is how you view yourself—not to mention how others view you, too. Take the time she was walking into a client's office. The people there hadn't seen her for a couple of weeks, and one employee said to another, "Who's that skinny woman over there?"

That exchange took place just 2 weeks after Guff started the Abs Diet—and she felt the effects immediately. Guff, 43, who runs marathons, has always been in good shape. But the effect of having two kids had taken a toll on her belly. "I was in pretty good shape, except for my stomach," she says. "But since going on the plan, I really noticed a difference. I could probably crunch walnuts with my abs."

The key for Guff was changing the way she approached eating. Sacrificing her own eating habits to get her kids out the door and keep up with her fitness training, she'd start the

cardiovascular fitness benefits. Second, circuit training keeps your workout short; you won't waste time resting between sets of an exercise, which means you can get on with the rest of your busy life.

Compound exercises. Another key part of the strength-training program is compound exercises; that is, exercises that call into play multiple muscle groups rather than just focusing on one. For example, with the Abs Diet Workout, we don't want you to exercise your chest, and then your shoulders, and then your triceps, and then your forearms. We want you to hit many different muscles at the same time and then get out of the gym. What's best is that workouts that build 2 to 3 pounds of lean muscle for women take only 20 minutes three times a week. Not only do compound exercises make your workout more fun and more challenging, they will also increase the demands on your muscles—even though you're not actually doing more work. (For instance, the squat hits a whopping 256 muscles with just one movement!) Greater muscle demand triggers your body to produce more human growth hormone—a potent fat burner.

---

day with tea—and often little else. "I used to go out and run without eating anything, and that was really stupid," Guff says. "I was horrified to learn the truth—that exercising on an empty stomach causes you to burn muscle, not fat." But the simple strategies of the Abs Diet changed all that. "Now I'm having smoothies for breakfast, and it's made me fitter and stoked up my energy," Guff says.

Guff says she couldn't do a program in which she'd have to count calories or weigh food. "What I love about the Abs Diet is the flexibility," she says. "All I have to remember is the catchy acronym—ABS DIET POWER—and I can remember the 12 powerfoods."

The results: Guff is leaner—and stronger. And she's also more con-

fident. "When women look at other women, they look at their boobs, their butts, and their waists—especially women who've had children. Every woman who's had a child cares about having a flat stomach."

But the true measure of her success came in the form of a pair of satin pants. Guff says, "They're kinda hot, but my stomach showed when I wore them. I have two kids, so I have no business flashing my midsection." But after two weeks on the plan, she decided to put them to the public test.

"All these people started complimenting me. A guy I went to college with said, 'Nice outfit.' My husband said I looked great," Guff says.

If the only weight you've ever picked up comes from lemon meringue pie and not in the gym, don't worry that you're not familiar with working with weights. You can start by lifting any amount of weight that you're comfortable with— whether it's a pair of light dumbbells or a couple of cans of beans (Powerfood!). Even if you start small, you'll grow stronger, start to build lean muscle, and keep your metabolism revved. As you progress, you'll build and burn more.

Focus on intensity. Time and time again, research has shown that higher-intensity workouts promote weight loss better than steady-state activities. In a Canadian study from Laval University, researchers measured differences in fat loss between two groups of exercisers following two different workout programs. The first group rode stationary bikes four or five times a week and burned 300 to 400 calories per 30- to 45-minute session. The second group did the same, but only one or two times a week, and they filled the rest of their sessions with short intervals of high-intensity cycling. They hopped on their stationary bikes and pedaled as quickly as they could for 30 to 90 seconds, rested, and then repeated the process several times per exercise session. As a result, they burned 225 to 250 calories while cycling, but they had burned more fat at the end of the study than the workers in the first group. In fact, even though they exercised less, their fat loss was nine times greater. Researchers said that the majority of the fat burning took place after the workout.

The Abs Diet Workout recommends that you add one simple interval workout per week to complement your strength training. These are workouts of traditional cardiovascular exercise (running, swimming, biking) in which you alternate between periods of high intensity and periods of rest. (I'll explain more about how to create an effective interval workout in the next chapter.)

If You Don't Already Exercise

THE BEST PART about the 6-week Abs Diet Workout is that, for the first 2 weeks at least, you don't actually have to exercise. If you're not doing anything right now, it's not critical that you start immediately. Instead, I want you to concentrate on acclimating your body and your schedule to the Abs Diet.

On the other hand, why wait to fire up your fat-burning mechanisms? If you want to start a light strength-training program, do this workout three times a week: Alternate between three sets of pushups (on your knees if you're unable to do them with straight legs at first) and three sets of squats with no weight. Both exercises use your body weight as resistance and will get your body accustomed to a strength-training program. Do 8 to 10 repetitions of pushups, followed by 15 to 20 repetitions of squats. When that becomes too easy, increase the repetitions of pushups, and hold on to some form of weight—light dumbbells are best—while doing squats. This light workout, especially in combination with 30 minutes of brisk walking, will really fire up your fat burners.

If You're Already in the Exercise Habit

MAYBE YOU LIFT weights once or twice a week. Maybe you run a few miles every morning. Maybe you're favored to win the gold in the decathlon this summer. I dunno. What I do know is that no matter what your workout is now, you're probably going to build more muscle and burn more fat if you switch to the Abs Diet Workout.

Even if your current exercise program has been working well for you, experts agree that mixing up your workout every month or so is the best way to maximize your results. That's because gains in strength and overall fitness come from challenging your body to perform in ways it's not used to. Performing the same workout over and over again doesn't train your body to reach its potential; it just trains your body to be really, really good at performing that one workout. So I want you to consider switching your current workout over to the Abs Diet Workout, at least for a few weeks. I guarantee the results you'll see will be astounding.

The New Abs Diet Workout: Suggested Weekly Schedule

YOU CAN MIX and match the different workouts to meet your lifestyle needs. When you construct your schedule, make sure to:

▶ Leave at least 48 hours between weight workouts of the same body parts. Your muscles need time to recover and repair themselves after a workout.

1 day each week to rest with no formal exercise.

m up for 5 minutes before starting to exercise, either through a ˍ ght jog, riding on a stationary bike, jumping rope, or doing slow jumping jacks.

The three components of your weekly schedule include:

1. Strength training: three times a week. These are total-body workouts with one workout that puts extra emphasis on your legs.

2. Additional cardiovascular exercise: optional, on non-strength-training days. Examples are cycling, running, swimming, walking, and using cardio machines. An interval workout is recommended for 1 day a week, and light cardiovascular exercise like walking is recommended for 2 of your 3 off days.

3. Abs exercises: twice a week. I recommend doing them before your strength training or interval workouts (more on abs exercises in Chapter 15).

Chapter 14

THE NEW ABS DIET WORKOUT

The Easiest, Most Effective Workout Plan Ever

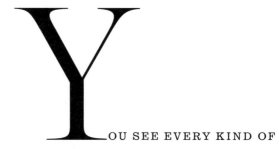OU SEE EVERY KIND OF person in the gym. The people with no fat. The people with no necks. The people with lots of fat. The people with lots of necks. And it seems they all get there a different way. I know that gym-goers have as many different workout philosophies as FOX has reality TV shows, but the one person I really know I can help is the overweight person who's working on tiny muscles in the corner. Working very small muscle groups—say, the one in your forearms or calves—is like putting on makeup before you take a shower. There's no point working on the fine points until you've taken care of the bigger issues.

That's why I've built a total-body strength training workout: to increase your lean muscle mass as efficiently as possible. It's simple: To show off your abs and flatten your belly, you have to burn fat. To burn fat, you have to build some muscle. Remember that adding just 1 pound of muscle will force your body to burn up to an additional 50 calories a day, every day.

This workout emphasizes the larger muscle groups of your body—chest, back, and legs. In one workout during the week, you'll give extra attention to your legs. I know what you're thinking: My abs are up here. Why do I care about working what's down there? Because most of your body's muscle is found below your belly button. Your lower body is where you'll build the most muscle in the least amount of time; working this giant muscle mass triggers the release of hormones that stimulate muscle growth throughout your body, kick your fat burners into overdrive, and give you that thin-as-a-dime stomach you want—in no time flat. Indeed, leg exercises are the key to total-body strength: In one Norwegian study, people who focused on lower-body work gained more upper-body strength than did those who emphasized upper-body exercises in their workouts. That doesn't mean you'll ignore your upper body entirely, though. With the upper-body workout, you'll also work your largest muscles—your chest, back, and shoulders—to burn more fat. If you follow this program, you'll still notice more growth and definition in your whole body—even your arms, even your shoulders, and yes, even your abs—and you'll begin to reshape your body.

Here, you're going to do circuit training to optimize your muscle-building potential. That is, you'll perform one set of an exercise and then move immediately to the next exercise, with just 30 seconds of rest. Follow the order of

||||||||||||||||||||||||||||||||||||||||||||||||||||||||||||||||||||||||||||||||||||||||||||||||

The Literally Last-Minute Weight-Loss Plan

Whether on the red carpet or at a photo shoot, models and actresses are used to showing lots of skin. Often, they'll use these last few tricks to make their bodies look their best. Here are instant ways to enhance and hone your appearance for the big day—whether it's at the beach or in a wedding gown.

Pump fast. Do quick strength moves like pushups or squats right before you show off. Increase your speed and reps in order to force blood into your muscles. More blood equals more tone.

Drink water. Guzzling a few glasses of H_2O before hitting the beach will help flush your system and relieve bloating.

Know your bloat foods. Avoid beans, for example, if they're hard for you to digest or if they make you bloat. Dairy has the same effect for some. And minimize your sodium intake. While there's no recommended dietary allowance, most nutritionists suggest you stay under 2,500 or 3,000 mg to avoid bloating (most of us have 5,000 milligrams a day).

the exercises I've listed on the following pages; that will allow you to work different body parts from set to set. (A complete set of exercise descriptions and instructional photos begins on page 190.) By alternating between body parts, you'll keep your body in constant work mode and be able to perform the movements back-to-back without rest. Here's why circuit training works so well: You'll save time because you'll cut the amount of rest you need when you alternate muscle groups. More important, you'll keep your heart rate elevated throughout the workout, so you'll burn even more fat while you're exercising— whether you're in the gym or in your own living room.

In the first 2 weeks of the program, do the circuit twice. Move from exercise to exercise with no more than 30 seconds of rest in between. When you complete one circuit, rest for 1 to 2 minutes, then complete the second circuit. After the first 2 weeks, when you've become comfortable doing two complete circuits during a workout, increase your workload to three circuits per workout. In every exercise, use a weight that you can handle comfortably for the number of repetitions noted. When that becomes too easy, increase the weight on each set by 10 percent or less. Here's a sample schedule of how you might arrange your workouts.

MONDAY:
Total-Body Strength Training Workout with Ab Emphasis
Complete one set of each ab exercise*, then complete the rest of the circuit twice.

EXERCISE	REPETITIONS	REST	SETS
Traditional Crunch*	12–15	none	1
Bent-Leg Knee Raise*	12–15	none	1
Oblique V-Up*	10 each side	none	1
Bridge*	1 or 2	none	1
Back Extension*	12–15	none	1
Squat	10–12	30 seconds	2
Bench Press	10	30 seconds	2
Pulldown	10	30 seconds	2
Military Press	10	30 seconds	2

(chart continues)

EXERCISE	REPETITIONS	REST	SETS
Upright Row	10	30 seconds	2
Triceps Pushdown	10–12	30 seconds	2
Leg Extension	10–12	30 seconds	2
Biceps Curl	10	30 seconds	2
Leg Curl	10–12	30 seconds	2

TUESDAY (OPTIONAL):
Light Cardiovascular Exercise Such as Walking
Try for 30 minutes at a brisk pace.

WEDNESDAY:
Total-Body Strength Training Workout with Ab Emphasis
Complete one set of each ab exercise*, then complete the rest
of the circuit twice.

EXERCISE	REPETITIONS	REST	SETS
Standing Crunch*	12–15	none	1
Pulse-Up*	12	none	1
Saxon Side Bend*	6–10 each side	none	1
Side Bridge*	1 or 2 each side	none	1
Back Extension*	12–15	none	1
Squat	10–12	30 seconds	2
Bench Press	10	30 seconds	2
Pulldown	10	30 seconds	2
Military Press	10	30 seconds	2
Upright Row	10	30 seconds	2
Triceps Pushdown	10–12	30 seconds	2
Leg Extension	10–12	30 seconds	2
Biceps Curl	10	30 seconds	2
Leg Curl	10–12	30 seconds	2

THURSDAY (OPTIONAL):
Light Cardiovascular Exercise Such as Walking
Try for 30 to 45 minutes at a brisk pace.

FRIDAY:
Total-Body Strength Training Workout with Leg Emphasis
Repeat entire circuit twice.

EXERCISE	REPETITIONS	REST	SETS
Squat	10–12	30 seconds	2
Bench Press	10	30 seconds	2
Pulldown	10	30 seconds	2
Traveling Lunge	10–12 each leg	30 seconds	2
Military Press	10	30 seconds	2
Upright Row	10	30 seconds	2
Step-Up	10–12 each leg	30 seconds	2
Triceps Pushdown	10–12	30 seconds	2
Leg Extension	10–12	30 seconds	2
Biceps Curl	10	30 seconds	2
Leg Curl	10–12	30 seconds	2

SATURDAY (OPTIONAL):
Abs Workout Plus Interval Workout
Complete one set of each ab exercise, then choose one interval workout from the selection on pages 212 and 215.

EXERCISE	REPETITIONS	REST	SETS
Traditional Crunch	12–15	none	1
Bent-Leg Knee Raise	12	none	1
Oblique V-Up	6–10 each side	none	1
Bridge	1 or 2	none	1
Back Extension	12–15	none	1

SUNDAY: OFF

Basic Exercises

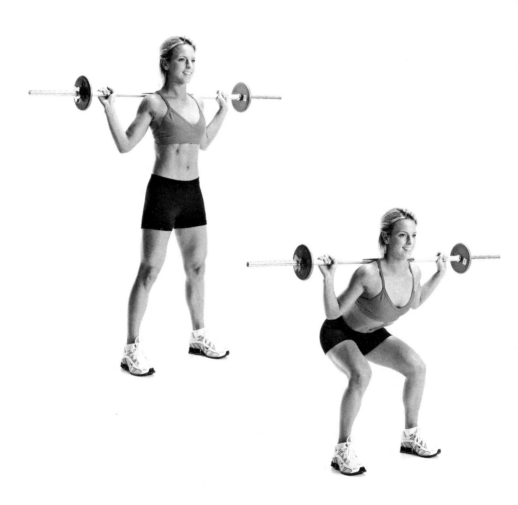

SQUAT

Hold a barbell with an overhand grip so that it rests comfortably on your upper back. Set your feet shoulder-width apart, and keep your knees slightly bent, back straight, and eyes focused straight ahead. Slowly lower your body as if you were sitting back into a chair, keeping your back in its natural alignment and your lower legs nearly perpendicular to the floor. When your thighs are parallel to the floor, pause, then return to the starting position.

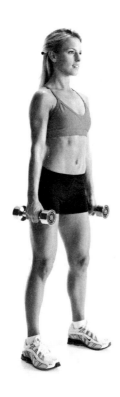

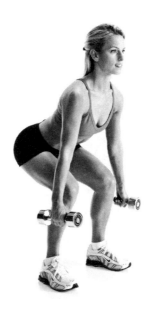

HOME VARIATION: *Same, but with one dumbbell in each hand, your palms facing your outer thighs.*

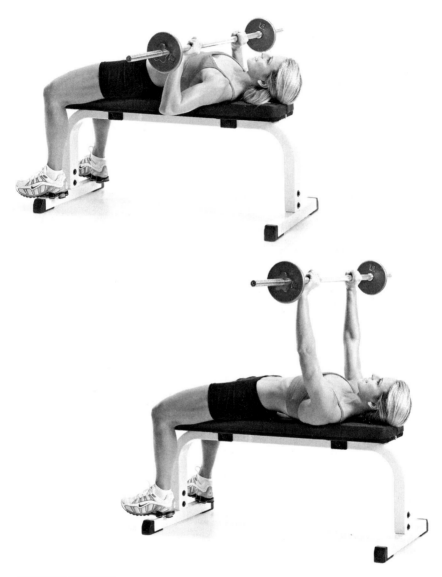

BENCH PRESS

Lie on your back on a flat bench with your feet on the floor. Grab the barbell with an overhand grip, your hands just beyond shoulder-width apart. Lift the bar off the uprights and hold it at arm's length over your chest. Slowly lower the bar to your chest. Pause, then push the bar back to the starting position.

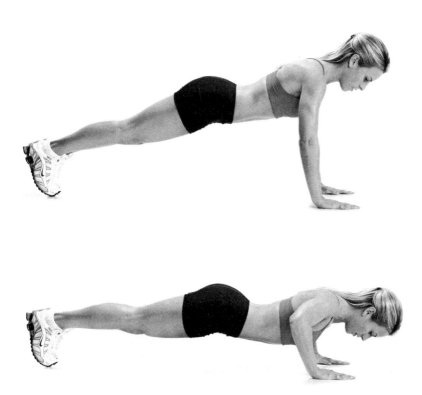

HOME VARIATION: *Just do standard pushups: Get in a pushup position with your hands about shoulder-width apart. Bend at the elbows while keeping your back straight, until your chin almost touches the floor, then push back up.*

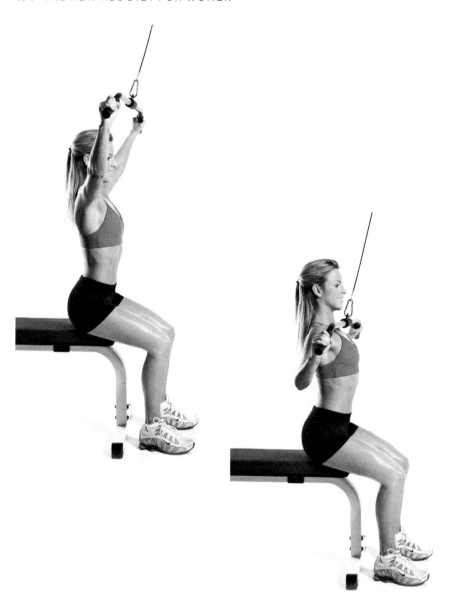

PULLDOWN

Stand facing a lat pulldown machine. Reach up and grasp the bar with an overhand grip that's 4 to 6 inches wider than your shoulders. Sit on the seat, letting the resistance of the bar extend your arms above your head. When you're in position, pull the bar down until it touches your upper chest. Hold this position for a second, then return to the starting position.

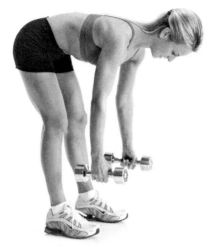

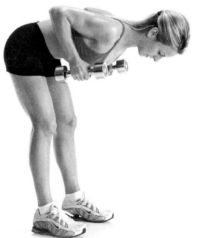

HOME VARIATION: *Bent-over row. Stand with your knees slightly bent and shoulder-width apart. Bend over so that your back is almost parallel to the floor. Holding a dumbbell in each hand, let your arms hang toward the floor. With your palms facing in, pull the dumbbells toward you until they touch the outside of your chest. Pause, then return to the starting position.*

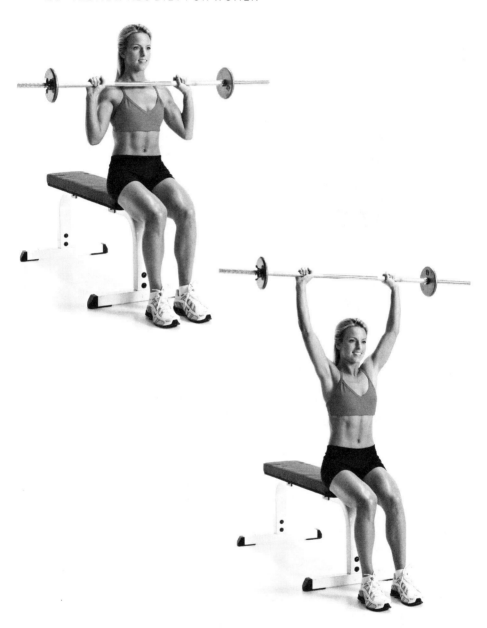

MILITARY PRESS

Sitting on an exercise bench, hold a barbell at shoulder height with your hands shoulder-width apart. Press the weight straight overhead so that your arms are almost fully extended, hold for a count of one, then bring it down to the front of your shoulders.

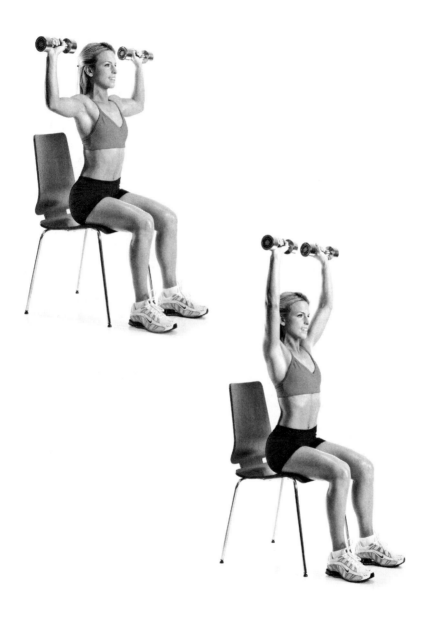

HOME VARIATION: *Sitting on a sturdy chair instead of a bench, hold one dumbbell in each hand, about level with your ears. Push the dumbbells straight overhead so that your arms are almost fully extended, hold for a count of one, then return to the starting position.*

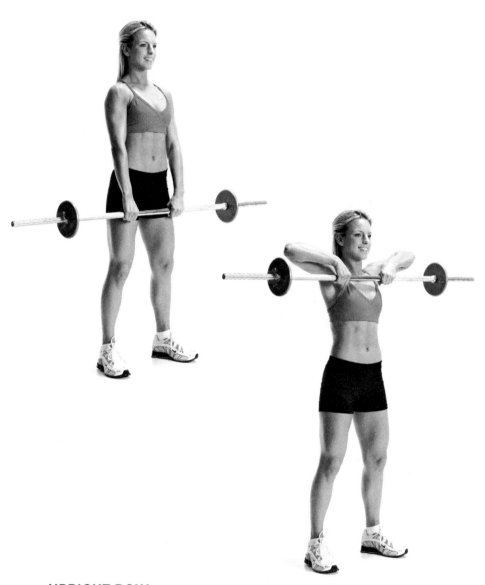

UPRIGHT ROW

Grab a barbell with an overhand grip, and stand with your feet shoulder-width apart and your knees slightly bent. Let the barbell hang at arm's length on top of your thighs, thumbs pointed toward each other. Bending your elbows, lift your upper arms straight out to the sides, and pull the barbell straight up until your upper arms are parallel to the floor and the bar is just below chin level. Pause, then return to the starting position.

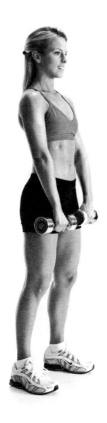

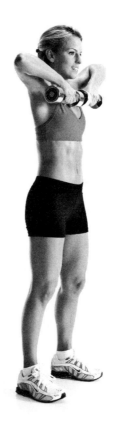

HOME VARIATION: *Same, using one dumbbell in each hand.*

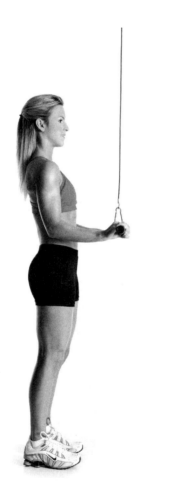
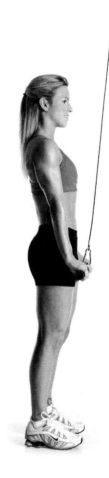

TRICEPS PUSHDOWN

While standing, grip a bar attached to a high pulley cable or lat machine with your hands about 6 inches apart. With your elbows tucked against your sides, bring the bar down until it is directly in front of you. With your forearms parallel to the floor (the starting position), push the bar down until your arms are extended straight down with the bar near your thighs. Don't lock your elbows. Return to the starting position.

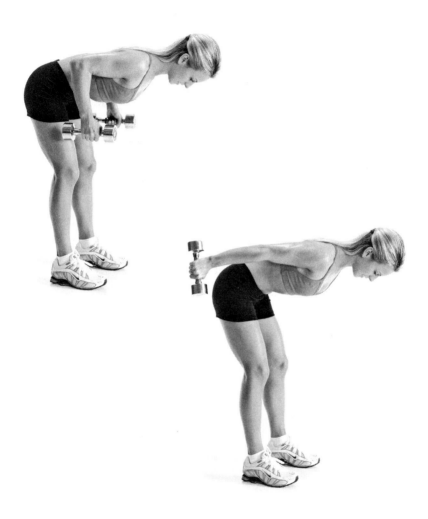

HOME VARIATION: *Triceps kickback. Stand with your knees slightly bent and shoulder-width apart. Bend over so that your back is almost parallel to the floor. Bend your elbows to about 90-degree angles, raising them to just above the level of your back. This is the starting position. Extend your forearms backward, keeping your upper arms stationary. When they're fully extended, your arms should be parallel to the ground. Pause, then return to the starting position.*

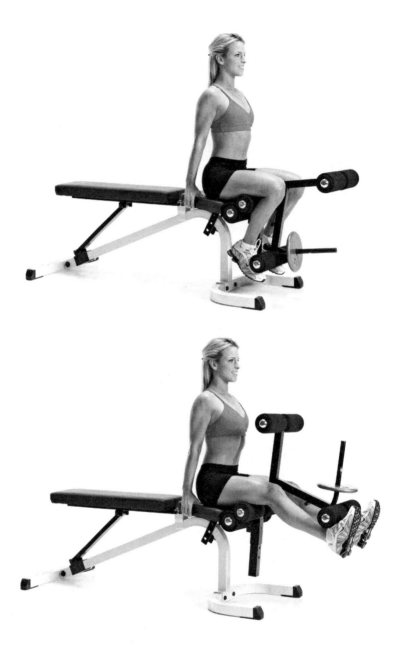

LEG EXTENSION

Sitting on a leg extension machine with your feet under the footpads, lean back slightly, and lift the pads with your feet until your legs are extended. Return to the starting position.

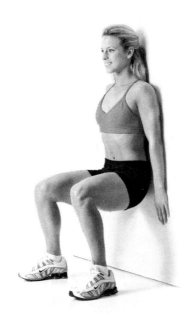

HOME VARIATION: *Wall squat. Stand with your back flat against a wall. Squat down so that your thighs are parallel to the ground. Hold that position for as long as you can. That's one set. Aim for 20 seconds to start and work your way up to 45 seconds. Return to the starting position.*

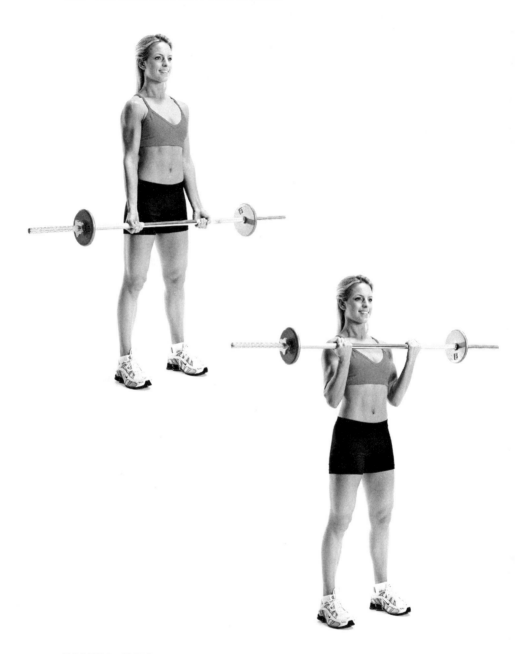

BICEPS CURL

Stand while holding a barbell in front of you, palms facing out, with your hands shoulder-width apart and your arms hanging in front of you. Curl the weight toward your shoulders, hold for a second, then return to the starting position.

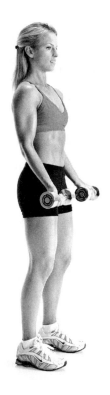

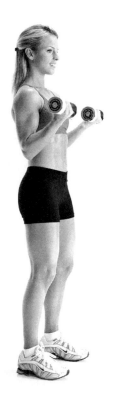

HOME VARIATION: *Same, only use a set of dumbbells instead.*

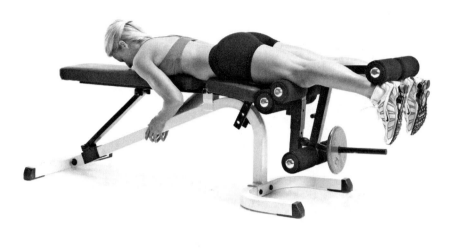

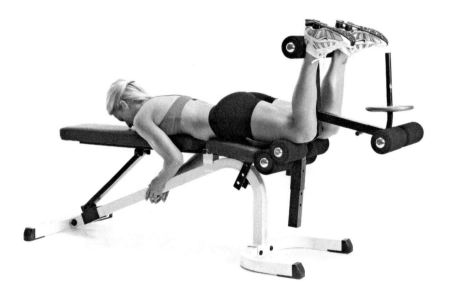

LEG CURL

Lie facedown on a leg curl machine and hook your ankles under the padded bar. Keeping your stomach and pelvis against the bench, slowly raise your feet toward your butt, curling up the weight. Come up so that your feet nearly touch your butt and slowly return to the starting position.

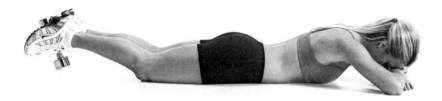

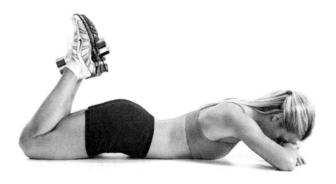

HOME VARIATION: *Lie down with your stomach on the floor. Put a light dumbbell between your feet (so that the top end of the dumbbell rests on the bottom of your feet). Squeeze your feet together and curl them up toward your butt. Slowly return to the starting position.*

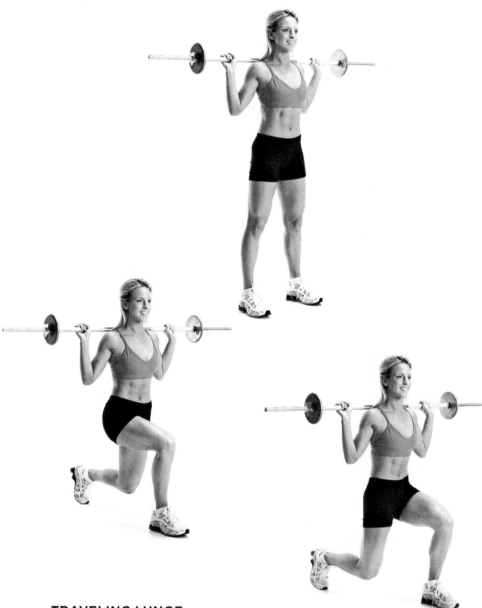

TRAVELING LUNGE

Rest a barbell across your upper back. Stand, with your feet hip-width apart, at one end of the room; you need room to walk about 20 steps. Step forward with your right foot and lower your body so that your right thigh is parallel to the floor and your left thigh is perpendicular to the floor (your left knee should bend and almost touch the floor). Stand and bring your left foot up next to your right, then repeat with the left leg lunging forward.

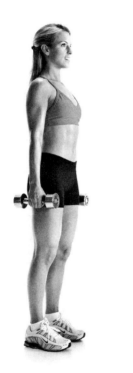

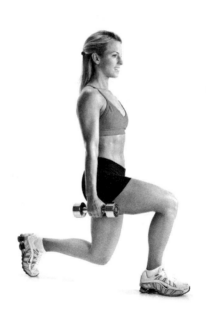

HOME VARIATION: *Use dumbbells, holding one in each hand with your arms at your sides. If you don't have enough space, do the move in one place, alternating your lead foot with each lunge.*

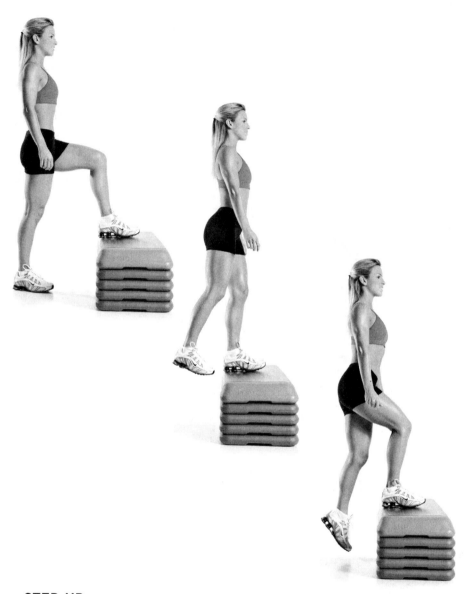

STEP-UP

Use a step or bench that's 18 inches off the ground. Place your left foot on the step so that your knee is bent at 90 degrees. Your knee should not advance past the toes of your left foot. Push off with your left foot and bring your right foot onto the step, keeping your back straight. Now step down with the left foot, followed by the right. Alternate the leading foot, or do all of the repetitions leading with one foot and then alternating. Once you're comfortable, add dumbbells.

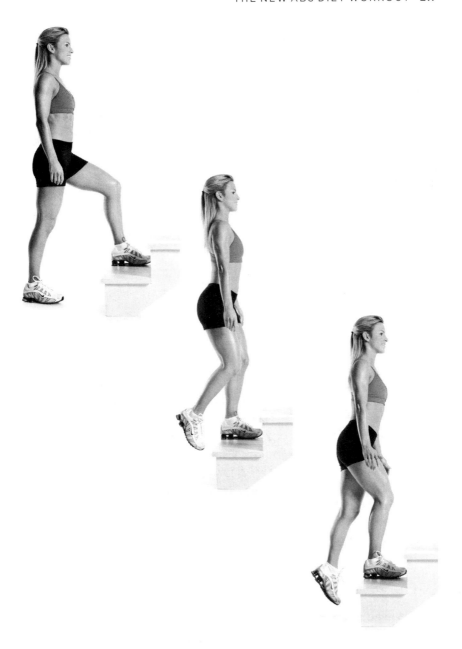

HOME VARIATION: *Same, only use a staircase instead of a step (if you don't have one).*

The New Interval Workouts

THEY SAY THAT slow and steady wins the race. But the cardiovascular key to fat burning is using interval workouts—workouts that alternate high-intensity levels with lower-intensity effort. Researchers in Canada found that exercisers who did 30-minute workouts that included short, hard bouts of effort lost three times as much fat in 15 weeks as their peers who performed 45-minute-long steady-paced, easier workouts. Interval training, the researchers determined, can increase your cells' ability to burn fat by up to 50 percent. What's more, intervals cause your body to burn calories long after you've stopped exercising. You can use intervals for running, cycling, swimming, on elliptical trainers, even walking if you alternate a speed walk and slow walk. To start, here are three new interval workouts.

Interval Variation I: The 20-Minute Sprinter

A typical interval: Switch between bouts of speed and 30-second recoveries.

> 5 minutes warmup (light jog, low intensity) or until you break a light sweat
>
> 10 seconds sprint pace (an 8 to 9 on an intensity scale of 1 to 10)
>
> 30 seconds recovery pace (about a 6 on that workout intensity scale)
>
> Repeat this sprint-recovery pattern for 10 minutes
>
> 5 minutes cooldown (starting at level 6 in intensity and gradually slowing down until you are walking during the last minute)
>
> Each week, increase the length of the sprint by 5 seconds until you are doing 30-second sprints and 30-second recoveries

Interval Variation II: The Pyramid

This pyramid structure allows you to step up to a long bout of peak effort in the middle of the workout and gradually come back down.

> 3–5 minutes warmup low intensity
>
> 30 seconds high intensity (7 to 8 on an intensity scale of 1 to 10)
>
> 1 minute low intensity (about a 4 in intensity)
>
> 45 seconds high intensity
>
> 1 minute low intensity

||||||||||||||||||||||||||||||||||||||||||||||||||||||||||||||||||||||||||||||||||||||||||||||||||||||

How to Improve Your Cardio Machine Workouts

Cardio machines help you work very hard in a very short period of time, making a morning or lunchtime workout an exercise in efficiency. But most people don't use the machines correctly. Fix your mistakes and you'll get more calorie burn for the effort.

EQUIPMENT	YOUR FORM	YOUR WORKOUT
Treadmill	**The mistake:** Too much bouncing up and down. Your head should remain relatively level while running, otherwise you'll tire out your joints—and yourself—too soon. **The fix:** Improve flexibility to smooth out your stride. Try leg swings—hold the handlebar, stand on one leg, and swing the other back and forth, keeping your upper body still. This will loosen your legs.	**The mistake:** Too many long, steady, flat runs. **The fix:** Run shorter and harder, mixing speeds and inclines to create intervals. Start with a 2 percent incline, and over several sessions work up to 10 percent. (Just walk at steep inclines.)
Stationary Bike	**The mistake:** The seat is too low or too high. A low seat fatigues the legs and stresses knees. Set it too high and your hips rock from side to side, which is inefficient. **The fix:** Adjust the seat, people! Sit on the seat and place your heel in the middle of the pedal, where the ball of your foot would normally go. You want your leg fully extended, at the lowest point of the pedal rotation. By moving your foot to the correct position on the pedal, you'll have the right amount of bend.	**The mistake:** Cruising instead of charging. **The fix:** Vary the intensity, with 2 to 3 minutes of high-cadence pedaling and a 3-minute recovery, then repeat for 15 minutes. Stand occasionally, which will add another dimension to your workout. Standing requires more muscle not only to push the pedals, but also to support and balance your body.

(chart continues)

EQUIPMENT	YOUR FORM	YOUR WORKOUT
Elliptical Trainer	**The mistake:** Too little resistance. Many people allow momentum to do the work for them instead of propelling the step with their leg muscles. **The fix:** Set the resistance correctly to be able to feel that you are pushing the ramp down when you make a revolution rather than flipping around freely.	**The mistake:** Getting bored. **The fix:** Do intervals. It will force you to reach a higher intensity of training for a sustained period of time. Try 90-second blasts every few minutes, with recoveries twice as long. Reduce recovery time as your fitness level increases.
Stair-climber	**The mistake:** Holding yourself up with your arms. A lot of people put their hands on the railing and lock their elbows with arms straight down. That's like using crutches. **The fix:** Rest your hands lightly on the bars only for balance. Keep your body upright, with just a slight lean forward.	**The mistake:** Too little resistance. **The fix:** Go slower, with challenging resistance. You'll give yourself a tougher workout, increase your heart rate and maintain your time in the training zone longer. **Result:** You'll burn more fat.
Rowing Machine	**The mistake:** Your hands bump your knees, which throws off your cadence. **The fix:** Take a tip from rowing crews to create a fluid motion: Think of the stroke as a dance, counting 1-2-3 and 3-2-1. On 1, push with your legs; on 2, "swing up" your body by leaning back; on 3, draw your arms to the bottom of your rib cage, spinning the flywheel. Then reverse it: 3, extend your arms; 2, swing your body forward from the hips; 1, bring your legs up after the handle passes your knees.	**The mistake:** A long, steady slog, which leads to inefficient exercise. You're spending too much time rowing at a moderate intensity. **The fix:** With medium resistance, do four to six 10-minute sets of high-intensity rowing with 2 to 3 minutes of rest in between. This will allow your heart rate to come down a bit so you can regroup with intense effort. **Result:** You'll expend more calories and get out of the gym quicker.

60 seconds high intensity

1 minute low intensity

90 seconds high intensity

1 minute low intensity

60 seconds high intensity

1 minute low intensity

45 seconds high intensity

1 minute low intensity

30 seconds high intensity

3–5 minutes cooldown low intensity, gradually slowing to a walk

Interval Variation III: 15-Minute Rope Burn

You remember skipping rope as a kid. Do you also remember how firm your calves and thighs were after a summer of double dutch jumping and *Strawberry Short-cake, Huckleberry Pie*? As you know, rope jumping takes a bit of coordination because you're using all your muscles and joints. That's also what makes it such a terrific calorie burner. And rope jumping is ideal for a fast, albeit tough, interval workout. Here's just one rope jumping interval. Make up more of your own.

5 minutes warmup (easy skipping)

30 seconds high intensity (80 percent of your maximum speed)

1 minute recovery (easy skipping)

30 seconds moderate intensity high-knee skips (lift your knees as high as you can while maintaining an even skip cadence)

1 minute recovery

Continue high-knee-skip-and-recovery pattern for two more circuits.

4 minutes alternate between skipping as fast as you can for 60 seconds and easy skipping for 60 seconds

60 seconds cool down (stop rope-skipping and walk for 2 minutes or until your heart rate returns to normal).

Customize the New Abs Diet Workout

YOU CAN MAKE some adjustments to the Abs Diet exercises and circuit, depending on your goals or how much time you have to exercise.

If your body type is lean and narrow: You want to build strength and curves with slow weight training. By lifting weight slowly, you'll challenge muscle fibers and help build them up faster—not to mention gaining some super muscle definition. Do the Abs Diet Circuit, but try doing each exercise with a slow, controlled movement. Try doing each repetition by taking 3 seconds to raise the weight and 3 seconds to lower it.

If your body is classically curvy: You want to balance and tone by burning fat and calories with a faster-paced routine. I recommend that you try the speed compound exercise superset starting on the next page.

If your body type is athletic: You want to get lean and energized with

|||||||||||||||||||||||||||||||||||||||||||||||||||||||||||||||||||||||||||||||||||||||||||||||||||||||

Dumbbell Smarts

When it comes to versatility, ease of use, and pure effectiveness, no muscle-building equipment beats dumbbells. On a practical level, they're inexpensive, indestructible, and compact. (Just try stuffing a Soloflex under the bed!) Eight reasons why smart folks surround themselves with dumbbells:

1. Dumbbells give you a more complete workout. You may think of dumbbells only in terms of biceps curls, but they're effective for working your legs (lunges, calf raises), back (deadlifts), and abdominals (side bends, weighted crunches) as well.

2. Dumbbells challenge your muscles more. When your body becomes used to a given workout, it stops being challenged, and your muscles stop growing. Because there are hundreds of different exercises you can do with dumbbells, you can keep updating your workout, so your muscles stay challenged—and keep growing.

3. Dumbbells build greater strength. Because they allow for a greater range of motion during exercise, dumbbells challenge your muscles in ways no other equipment can. For example, a barbell becomes restricting during a bench press because you can bring the weight down only so far before your chest gets in the way. But when you're holding a dumbbell in each hand, you can bring the weight down lower during each repetition, calling into play more muscle fiber and stimulating more growth.

4. Dumbbells build strength faster. Negative resistance training refers to the stress you put on your muscles during the lowering, or negative, phase of an exercise. And studies suggest that negative resistance may grow muscle even more effectively than the positive, or lifting, phase of an exercise. With dumbbells, you can add extra negative resistance into your workout. Let's say you've done 10 biceps curls with your left hand, and you can't possibly lift the weight one more time.

the active yoga, dance, and Pilates postures that you will find beginning on page 323. These exercises will help you maintain and tone your athletic build.

Tone Your Body Twice as Fast
with Compound Exercises

SOMETIMES YOU JUST can't spare 30 minutes for a workout. You have 10, maybe, tops. It's times like these when compound moves can help you stay true to your program. Compound exercises combine two different moves into one so you can work multiple muscle groups in 1 set. For example, the dumbbell thruster on

||||||||||||||||||||||||||||||||||||||||||||||||||||||||||||||||||||||||||||||||||||||||||||||||||||||||||||||||||||||||||||||||

You can now use your right hand to help your left lift the weight one more time, and simply lower the dumbbell using your left hand only. This helps you squeeze out that last little bit of benefit from your workout.

5. Dumbbells can give you a healthier heart. Plenty of studies have shown that weight training reduces blood pressure and indirectly strengthens the heart. Researchers have also shown that a dumbbell workout can yield additional benefits, including a lower lipid profile (less gum for your arteries) and increased oxygen uptake. Dumbbells do a better job at this than other weight-training equipment, again because of the greater range of motion they allow.

6. Dumbbells make you work in three dimensions: They don't lock you into the up-and-down or side-to-side motions that exercise machines do. That means your muscles learn to function well in real life, whether you're catching a Frisbee at the beach or catching the kids before they fall off the swings.

7. Dumbbells keep your body in balance. By forcing each arm to lift its fair share, dumbbells help to immediately identify strength imbalances that may have developed from sports, from simple acts like driving or carrying a briefcase, or from lifting with barbells or machines. When pressing a barbell overhead, for example, you can compensate for a weaker left arm by pushing more with your right side—and just make the imbalance worse. When you're pressing two dumbbells overhead, however, each side of your body has to work independently—and each side gets the same amount of exercise.

8. Dumbbells help prevent injury. While exercise machines are calibrated to target one muscle exclusively, dumbbells strengthen you everywhere, especially in your body's important but often overlooked small muscles, ligaments, and tendons. Machines may miss these, setting you up for injury.

page 220, combines a squat with an overhead press, working the shoulders as well as the legs in one efficient sequence. Now, if you pair two compound moves into a superset, you'll double the intensity of the set and significantly boost your calorie burn. Take a look at the total-body combinations on the following pages and use them to avoid skipping your workout when your day is crazy busy. Do 6 to 10 repetitions of each pair of combination exercises, for example, the deadlift and bent-over row combo and the Swiss-ball pike with pushup. Rest for 90 seconds after finishing both. Then move to the next pair of combo moves, and so on, resting 90 seconds between supersets. The total workout should take you less than 15 minutes. When you have more time, do 2 sets of each superset. Really strapped for time? Choose any pair of combo moves and perform 3 sets without any rest.

llllllllllllllllllllllllllllllllllllllllllllllllllllllllllllllllllllllllllllllllllllllllllllllllllllll

The 10-Minute Total-Body Dumbbell Pump

When you don't have time for a longer workout, try this super-fast dumbbell combination lift. It works every major muscle group in one fast and furious circuit. Do 2 to 3 sets of 12 repetitions, and you're done for the day.

Warmup: Start by doing 5 minutes of calesthenics (jumping jacks, bodyweight squats, rope jumping, whatever you wish) to warm up your muscles.

Step 1: Grab a pair of lightweight dumbbells and get into a pushup position, with your arms straight and directly beneath your shoulders and your hands on the dumbbells. Use hexagonal dumbbells, so they won't roll when you do the pushup.

Step 2: Do a pushup. Then bring your feet underneath you, one foot at a time.

Step 3: Keeping your back flat, stand up. (This is a deadlift.)

Step 4: From the standing position, curl the weights up to your shoulders.

Step 5: Swing your elbows out to your sides so that the weights are above your shoulders. Lower your body until your thighs are parallel to the floor. Pause, then stand up as you press the weights overhead. (This combines a weighted squat with an overhead press.)

Step 6: Lower the weights to your sides. Bend your knees, place the dumbbells on the floor shoulderwidth apart and get back into pushup position with your hands on the dumbbells. Now repeat the steps for a total of 10 repetitions.

Compound Exercises for Quick Workouts
Superset 1

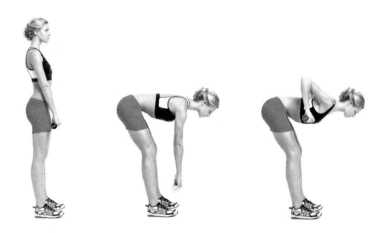

BENT-OVER ROW AND DEADLIFT COMBO

Stand with your feet hip-width apart, holding dumbbells at your thighs. Keeping your knees bent slightly, bend at the waist until your torso is parallel to the floor. Pause, then pull the weights up toward your rib cage. Lower them, press back on your heels, and stand. That's 1 repetition.

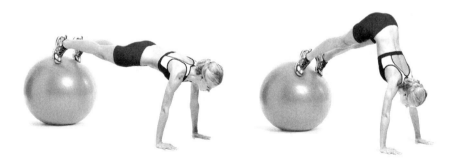

SWISS-BALL PIKE WITH PUSHUP

Start in a pushup position with your toes on a stability ball and your hands on the floor. Keeping your legs straight, raise your butt toward the ceiling, drawing the ball toward your arms. Pause and roll back to the starting position. Pause, then do a pushup. That's 1 repetition.

Superset 2

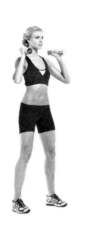 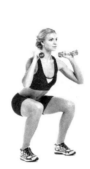 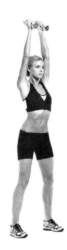

THRUSTER

Hold a pair of dumbbells just above your shoulders. Bend your knees into a squat, until your thighs are parallel to the floor. Push yourself up, pressing the weights straight up as you stand. Pause, then lower them to your shoulders. That's 1 repetition.

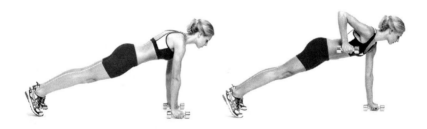

PUSHUP ROW WITH CORE HOLD

Get into pushup position with your arms straight and your hands resting on dumbbells, feet slightly wider than hip-width apart. Brace your abs as you pull one dumbbell toward your body until your elbow is above your back. Pause, then slowly return the weight to the floor and repeat with the other arm. That's 1 repetition.

Superset 3

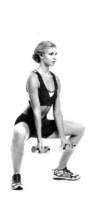
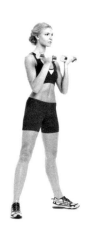

SUMO SQUAT AND CURL

Stand with your feet wider than hip-width apart, toes turned out, holding a pair of dumbbells between your knees. This is the start. Bending at your knees, lower your body until your thighs are parallel with the floor. Push yourself back up as you curl the weights up to your shoulders. Return to start. That's 1 repetition.

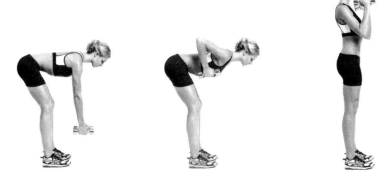

ROW AND BACK EXTENSION

Stand with your feet hip-width apart, holding a pair of dumbbells in front of you. Keeping your knees slightly bent, lean forward at the waist until your torso is parallel to the floor and the weights are at mid-shin level. This is the starting position. Pull the weights up toward your rib cage. Stand up, holding the dumbbells at your shoulders. Reverse the movements by lowering to the bent-over row position and extending your arms back to the starting position. That's 1 repetition.

Superset 4

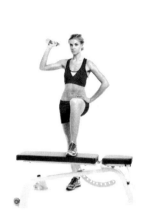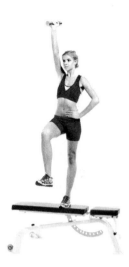

STEP-UP AND SINGLE-ARM PRESS

Hold a dumbbell in your right hand with your upper arm parallel to the floor and place your left foot on a step or bench. Lift yourself onto the step as you press the weight over your shoulder. Lower both back to the starting position. That's 1 rep. Finish all the reps with your left leg and right arm, then repeat with your right leg and left arm.

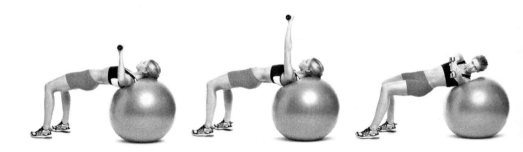

DUMBBELL PRESS AND CORE ROLL

Holding a dumbbell at your left shoulder, lie on a stability ball, keeping your hips in line with your knees. Push the dumbbell straight up to full extension. Grab your left wrist and rotate your body to the left, keeping your hips in position. Return your shoulders to the ball and lower the weight to your shoulder. That's 1 rep. Finish the reps on the left, then repeat the exercise while holding the dumbbell in your right hand.

Chapter 15

TARGETING YOUR ABS
A 50-"Six-Pack" of Exercises

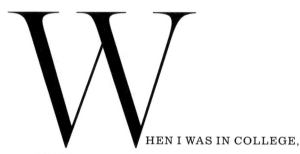

HEN I WAS IN COLLEGE, I had a friend who argued that he knew the key to a six-pack: "All you have to do is 1,000 crunches a day for a month." He said it in a way that made you believe him—that if only you were disciplined enough to put in the time every day to concentrate on your abdominal muscles, then you'd eventually chisel away a gut of stone. His theory was that it all boiled down to volume and discipline. He went on to say that the iconic ab exercise would do more than just build abs—that it was also the fix-all to weight problems, that you could simply crunch away years of bingeing on pizza, fries, and ranch dressing by the gallon.

In a lot of ways (a heck of a lot of ways, actually), my friend was wrong. For one, crunching won't burn fat. And you won't develop abs by doing the same exercise over and over—let alone the same exercise every day. And 1,000 repetitions? C'mon. There's only one thing many of us would do 1,000 times a day if it were physically possible, and it wouldn't be a crunch. But he was right in one sense: If you want abs that will make you stronger, healthier, and better looking, you do have to work them. And that does take some discipline—but not as much as you'd think.

Though your midsection works as one unified core, it does help to think of your abdominal center in regions. To build a defined belly, you need to work the entire region. The three visible regions consist of the upper abs, lower abs, and obliques (the muscles along the side of your torso). But there are also a number of supporting muscles that, when developed, will add strength to your abdominals: your lower back and the transverse abdominis—muscles that run underneath your abdomen horizontally to give support to your entire midsection.

‖‖

Reacquaint Yourself with Your Abs

Your abdominal muscles are a lot like a skilled group of employees. The harder they work, the better they make you look, and vice versa.

This is because you use your abs in virtually every movement that matters. Lifting. Running. Jumping. Reproducing. (It takes a lot of midsection stability to stand over that copy machine. Especially when it's printing on both sides of the page.) So the stronger they are, the harder and longer you'll be able to play. Here's a quick course in the anatomy of your abs.

Rectus abdominis. This is the six-pack muscle that helps your upper body bend (like in a crunch) and also helps keep good posture. It's what people think of when they think of abs.

External obliques. These muscles start on the ribs and extend diagonally down the sides of your waist. If a movement happens at your waist, the external obliques are involved. The torso rotation that's key to golf, tennis, and hockey is mostly a function of the external obliques. Even the basic crunching motion, attributed to the rectus abdominis (the six-pack muscle), wouldn't be possible without a strong contraction of the external obliques to stabilize the torso.

Internal obliques. These lie between the rib cage and the external obliques and also extend diagonally down the sides of your waist. Similar to the externals, the internal obliques are involved in torso rotation. You use these muscles when you breathe deeply.

Transverse abdominis. It's a thin muscle that runs horizontally, surrounding your abdomen. It's also known as the girdle because it functions as a compressor for the abdomen, keeping everything in place.

You already have all of these muscles; you just need them to come front and center. That's why your priorities have to revolve around the first two components: the nutrition principles and the fat-burning workout. Once you strip away the fat, your abs can grow and show. Unlike what my friend said, you won't get a six-pack by working your abdominal muscles every day. Instead, follow these guidelines for adding the final component.

Work your abdominals just 2 or 3 days a week. Don't make the common mistake of overtaxing them in hopes of speeding results. Abs are like any other muscle in your body. They'll grow when they're at rest, not when you're working them. So working them every day doesn't give them a chance to grow and get strong. You will develop abs by working them two or three times a week. I'd recommend adding the ab circuit to the beginning of your workout. Saving them until the end of the workout means there's more possibility that you'll skimp and take shortcuts.

Hit the whole region, not just the famed rectus abdominus. (See "Reaquaint Yourself with Your Abs.") You have five regions that you're going to work: your upper abs, lower abs, obliques, transverse abdominis, and your lower back muscles. These muscle regions form the spine-supporting girdle of muscle that makes up what's called your core. For each workout, pick one exercise per region to ensure that you're hitting every core muscle group.

Pick different exercises every workout. We're giving you a huge selection of exercises for your abdominals, but you need to pick only five exercises for each workout. The key is variety: Changing your routine doesn't allow your abs to get comfortable, which means they'll continue to grow after each workout.

Do a circuit. In the first week of workouts, just do 1 set of each exercise (10 to 15 repetitions, depending on the exercise). In the 2nd and 3rd weeks, do 2 sets if you'd like, but perform them in a circuit so that you're doing each exercise once before repeating an exercise. After that, you can do three circuits. Even then, your ab workouts shouldn't take more than 5 minutes.

Go slow. Each rep of an ab exercise should last slightly longer than Kajagoogoo lasted on the radio—4 to 6 seconds. Any faster, and you run the risk of letting momentum do the work. The slower you go, the higher the intensity. The higher the intensity, the stronger the stomach.

Remember that this portion of the workout is what will make your belly as tight as a size-too-small pair of high heels. Think of the ab exercise portion of the plan as the toy at the bottom of the cereal box, the paycheck at the end of the week, the finish line at the end of the marathon. It's the motivation. It's the reward. It's the goal that no scale could ever show.

How to Do the Workout

PICK ONE EXERCISE from each group of the listings below and do the exercise for the specified number of repetitions. Do 1 set of each exercise, and then repeat the circuit.

Note: Many of these exercises target different regions of the abdominals during the same movement, but they're grouped based on what areas they primarily target. They've also been grouped by levels of difficulty so that you can change your workouts as you get stronger. For each exercise, pause at the end of the movement and return to the starting position. That counts as one repetition, unless otherwise noted.

The Abs Circuit

Upper Abs (pages 227 to 236)

Lower Abs (pages 237 to 246)

Obliques (pages 247 to 252)

Transverse Abdominis (pages 253 to 260)

Lower Back (pages 261 to 264)

Upper Abs

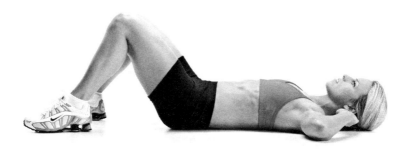

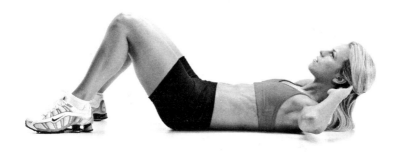

TRADITIONAL CRUNCH

Lie on your back with your knees bent and your hands behind your ears.
Slowly crunch up, bringing your shoulder blades off the ground.

12 to 15 repetitions [*Beginner*]

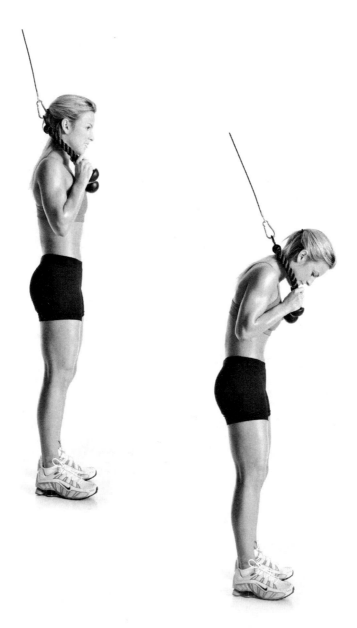

STANDING CRUNCH

Attach a rope handle to a high cable pulley. Stand with your back to the weight stack and hold the ends of the rope behind your head. Crunch down.

12 to 15 repetitions [*Beginner*]

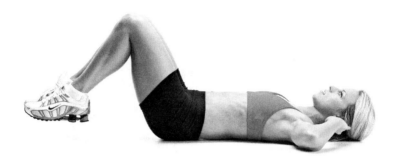

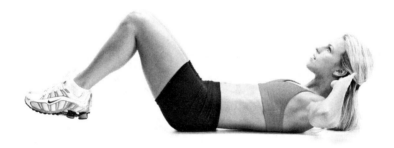

MODIFIED RAISED-FEET CRUNCHES

Lie on your back with your knees bent and your hands behind your ears. Raise your feet just a few inches off the floor and hold them there. Crunch up, then lower your torso back to the floor, keeping your feet raised throughout the movement.

12 to 15 repetitions [*Beginner to intermediate*]

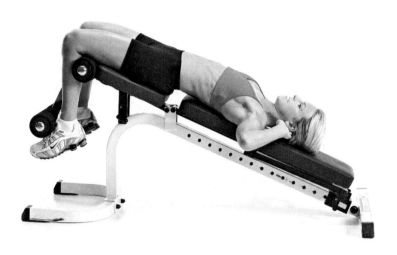

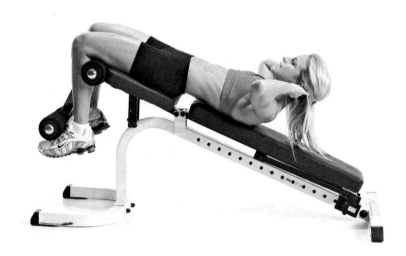

DECLINE CRUNCH

Lie on your back on a decline board, with your ankles locked under the padded support bars and your fingertips cupped behind your ears. Lift your shoulder blades off the bench, keeping your lower body flat. Don't jerk your body to build momentum. Hold the contraction for a second.

12 to 15 repetitions [*Beginner to intermediate*]

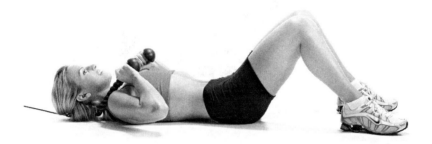

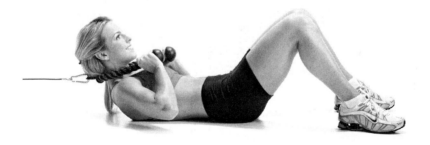

LYING CABLE CRUNCH

Attach a rope handle to the low pulley. Lie on the floor with your head near the low pulley, your knees bent, and your feet flat on the floor. Hold the handle over your chest so that the point of the rope attachment is at the base of your neck. Crunch your rib cage toward your pelvis, lifting your shoulder blades a few inches off the floor.

12 to 15 repetitions [*Intermediate to advanced*]

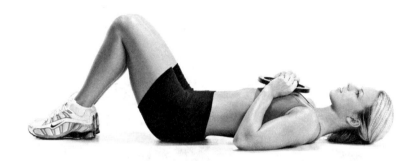

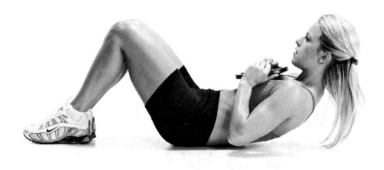

WEIGHTED CRUNCH

Lie on your back with your knees bent, holding a weight plate or dumbbell across your chest. Slowly crunch up, bringing your shoulder blades off the ground. Use progressively heavier weight.

12 to 15 repetitions [*Intermediate to advanced*]

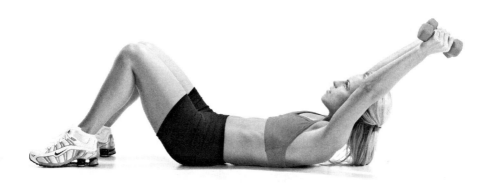

LONG-ARM WEIGHTED CRUNCH

Lie on your back with your knees bent. Hold a light dumbbell in each hand and stretch your arms straight back behind you. Crunch your rib cage toward your pelvis. Don't generate momentum with your arms.

12 to 15 repetitions [*Intermediate to advanced*]

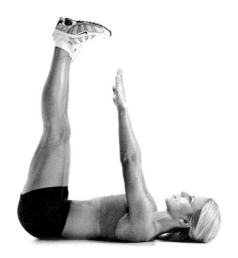

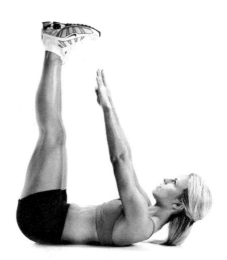

TOE TOUCH

Lie on your back with your legs raised directly over your hips; your knees should
be slightly bent. Raise your arms straight up, pointing toward your toes, and relax
your head and neck. Use your upper abs to raise your rib cage toward your pelvis,
lift your shoulder blades off the floor, and reach toward your toes. Hold for a second.
Lower your shoulders to the floor and repeat.

12 to 15 repetitions [*Intermediate to advanced*]

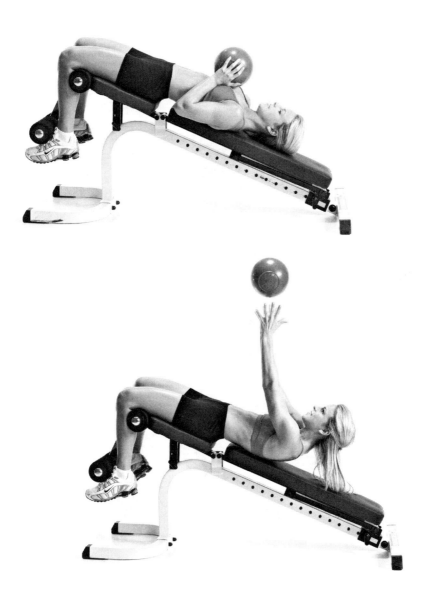

MEDICINE BALL BLAST

Set an adjustable ab bench at a 45-degree angle. Lie down on it with your head toward the floor and hook your feet under the padded support bars. Hold a medicine ball at your chest as you lower yourself. As you come up, chest-pass the ball straight up over your head. Catch it at the top of the movement, then lower yourself and repeat.

12 to 15 repetitions [*Advanced*]

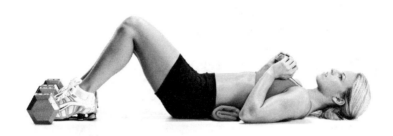

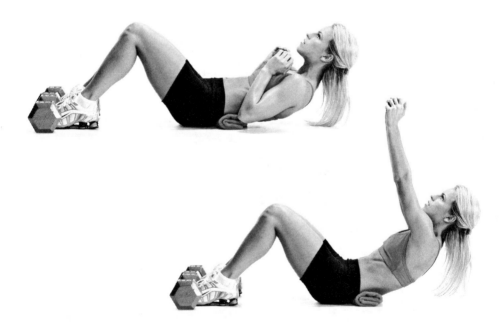

SICILIAN CRUNCH

Slide your feet under the handles of heavy dumbbells. Place a rolled-up towel under your lower back and hold a dumbbell across your chest. Raise your upper body as high as possible by crunching your rib cage toward your pelvis. At the top of the move, straighten your arms and raise the dumbbell above your head. Keep the dumbbell above your head and take 4 seconds to lower your body to the starting position.

10 repetitions [*Advanced*]

Lower Abs

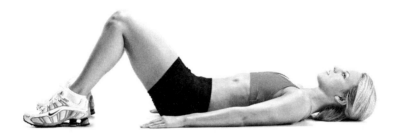

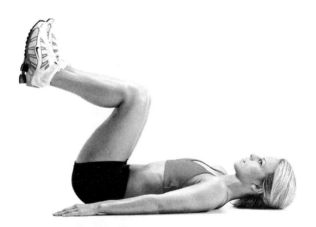

BENT-LEG KNEE RAISE

Lie on your back with your head and neck relaxed and your hands on the floor near your butt. Your feet should be flat on the floor. Use your lower abdominal muscles to raise your knees up toward your rib cage, then slowly lower your feet back to the starting position. As your feet lightly touch the floor, repeat.

12 repetitions [*Beginner*]

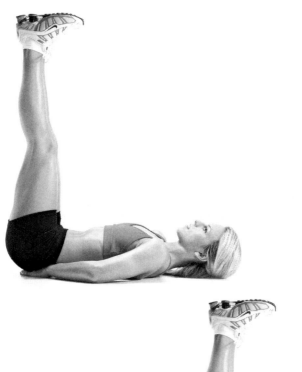

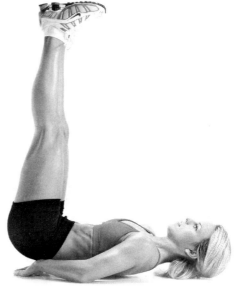

PULSE-UP

Lie with your hands underneath your tailbone and your legs raised and pointed straight up toward the ceiling, perpendicular to your torso. Pull your navel inward and flex your glutes as you lift your hips just a few inches off the floor. Then lower your hips.

12 repetitions [*Beginner*]

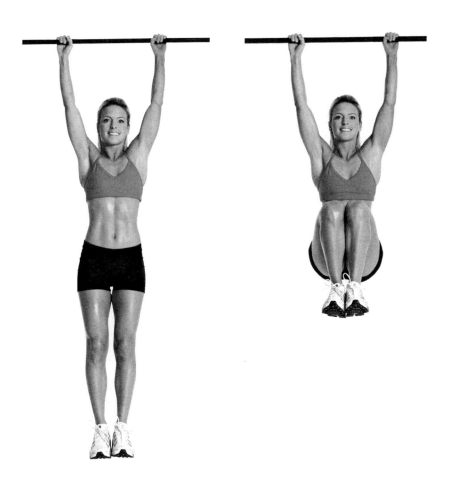

HANGING KNEE RAISE

Hang fully extended from a chinup bar, with your palms facing out and your hands a little farther than shoulder-width apart. (Your feet may lightly touch the floor.) Raise your knees toward your chest, curling your pelvis upward at the end. When you can do that for 12 repetitions, make it tougher by keeping your legs straight instead of bending your knees or by holding a medicine ball between your knees.

12 repetitions [*Beginner to intermediate*]

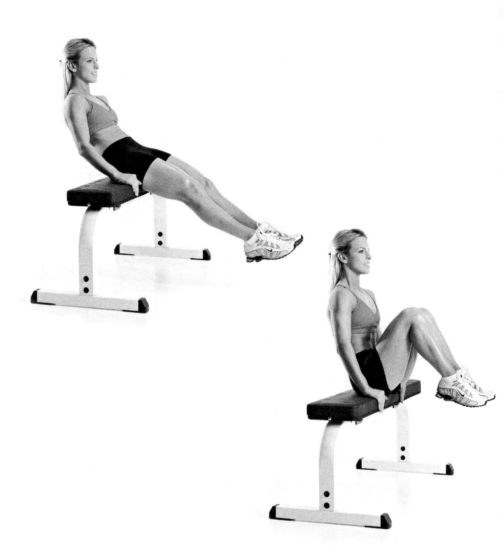

SEATED AB CRUNCH

Sit on the edge of a stable chair or bench. Place your hands in front of your butt and grip the sides of the seat. Lean back slightly and extend your legs down and away, keeping your heels 4 to 6 inches off the floor. To begin the exercise, bend your knees and slowly raise your legs toward your chest. At the same time, lean forward with your upper body, allowing your chest to approach your thighs.

12 repetitions [*Beginner to intermediate*]

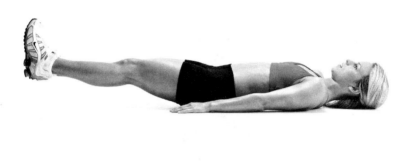

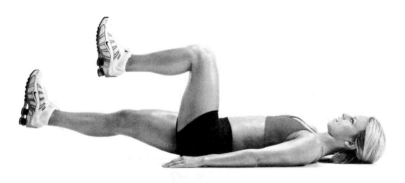

RAISED KNEE-IN

Lie on your back. Your arms should be close to your sides, with your palms down and just under your lower back and butt. Press the small of your back against the floor and extend your legs outward, with your heels about 3 inches above the floor. Keeping your lower back against the floor, lift your left knee toward your chest. Your right leg should remain hovering above the floor. Hold, then straighten your left leg to the starting position and repeat with your right leg. Keep your abs tight throughout the exercise.

8 to 12 repetitions each side [*Intermediate*]

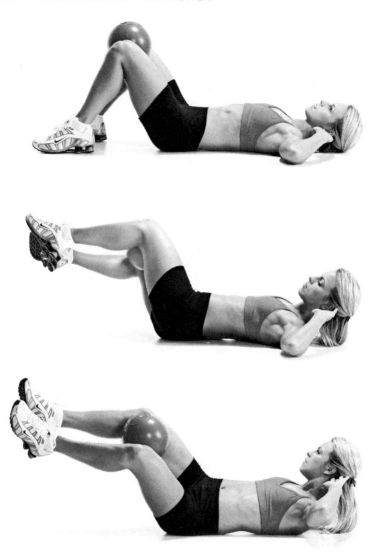

FIGURE-8 CRUNCH

Lie on your back with your knees bent at a 90-degree angle and your feet flat on the floor. Squeeze a light medicine ball tightly between your knees. Cup your hands lightly over your ears, then slowly raise your head, shoulders, and feet off the floor. Move your knees in a wide figure-8 motion. Do three repetitions in one direction, then reverse the motion for 3 repetitions.

6 repetitions [*Intermediate*]

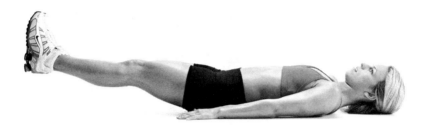

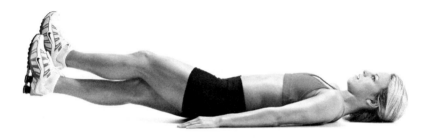

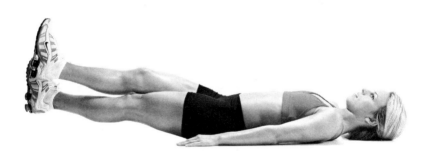

FLUTTER KICK

Lie on your back, raise both feet about a foot off the ground, and scissor-kick one leg over the other.

20 repetitions [*Intermediate*]

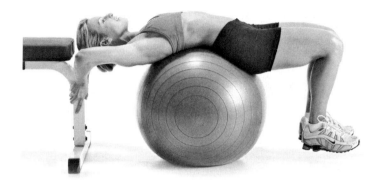

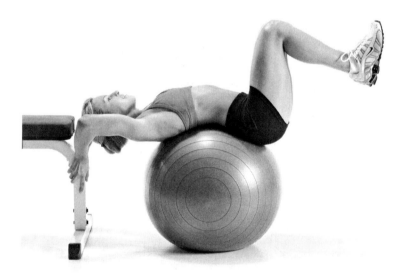

SWISS BALL KNEE RAISE

Lie faceup on a Swiss ball, with your hips lower than your shoulders. Reach back and grab something that won't move, such as a bench or desk. Lift and bend your legs so that your feet are off the floor and the lower parts of your legs point ahead. (To make it more difficult, hold your legs straight out.) Do a standard Bent-Leg Knee Raise, using your abs and hip flexors to curl your knees toward your chest.

12 repetitions [*Intermediate to advanced*]

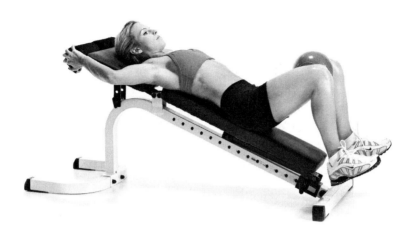

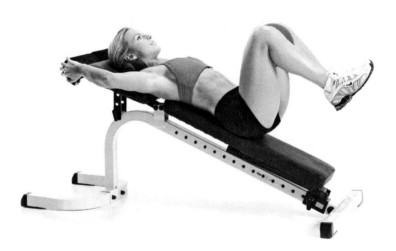

REVERSE CRUNCH HOLDING MEDICINE BALL

Lie on a slant board with your hips lower than your head. Grab the bar behind your head for support. Bend your hips and knees at 90-degree angles and hold a small medicine ball between your knees. Start with your butt flat against the board. Pull your hips up and in toward your rib cage. Curl them as high as you can without lifting your shoulders off the board, and keep your hips and knees at 90-degree angles.

12 repetitions [*Intermediate to advanced*]

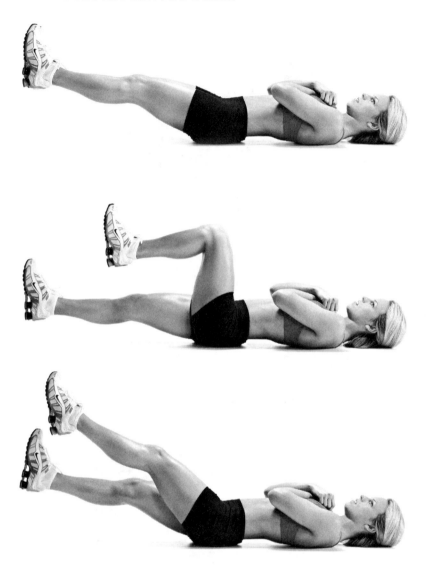

PUSH-AWAY

Lie on your back with your hands on your chest, legs extended, feet raised off the floor.
Alternately bring each knee toward your head, then forcefully kick forward. Don't let
your feet touch the floor. (If you feel any discomfort in your lower back while performing this exercise, try lifting your head and tucking your chin toward your chest.)

10 repetitions each side [*Intermediate to advanced*]

Obliques

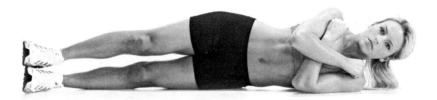

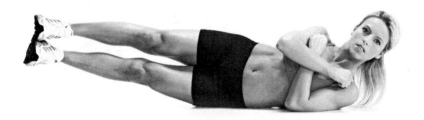

OBLIQUE V-UP

Lie on your side with your body in a straight line. Fold your arms across your chest. Keeping your legs together, lift them off the floor as you raise your top elbow toward your hip. The range of motion is short, but you should feel an intense contraction in your obliques.

10 repetitions each side [*Beginner*]

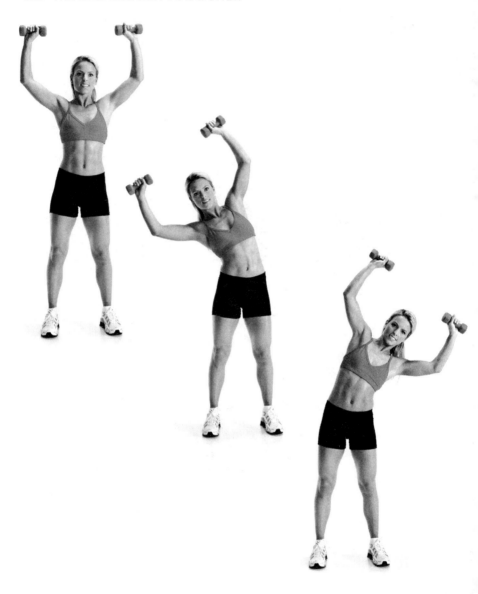

SAXON SIDE BEND

Hold a pair of lightweight dumbbells over your head, in line with your shoulders, with your elbows slightly bent. Keep your back straight, and slowly bend directly to your right side as far as possible without twisting your upper body. Pause, return to an upright position, then bend to your left side as far as possible.

6 to 10 repetitions each side [*Beginner to intermediate*]

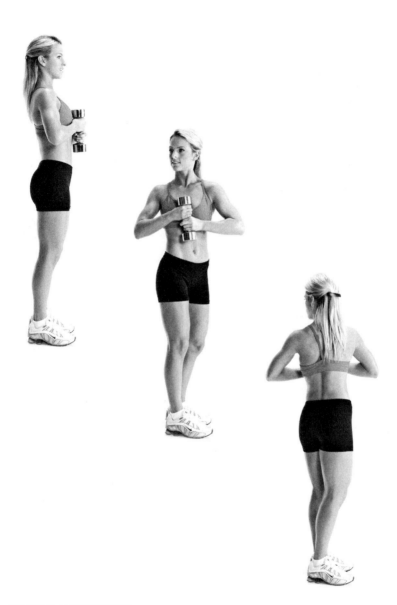

SPEED ROTATION

Stand while holding a dumbbell with both hands in front of your midsection.
Twist 90 degrees to the right, then 180 degrees to your left. Keep your abs tight
and move fast. Bring to center. Alternate the side you start with.

10 repetitions each side [*Intermediate*]

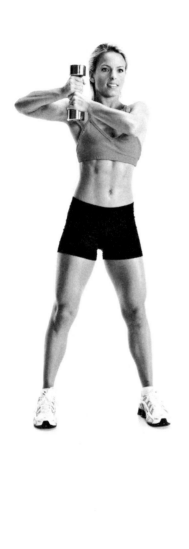

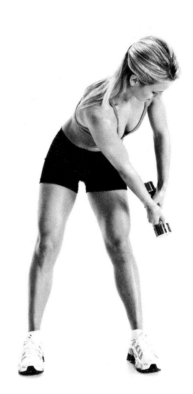

TWO-HANDED WOOD CHOP

Stand while holding a dumbbell, with both hands next to your right ear. Flex your abs
and rotate your torso to the left as you extend your arms and lower the dumbbell to
the outside of your left knee. Lift it back, finish the set, and repeat on the other side.

10 repetitions each side [*Intermediate*]

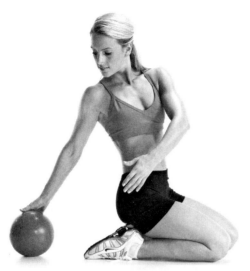

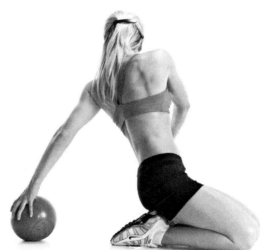

MEDICINE BALL TORSO ROTATION

Hold a medicine ball or basketball in front of you. Sit with your knees bent and your feet on the floor. Quickly twist to your left and set the ball behind your back. Twist to the right and pick up the ball. Bring the ball around to your left and set it down again. Repeat. Do the same number of repetitions in which you first twist to the left side as you do when you twist to the right side.

10 repetitions each side [*Intermediate to advanced*]

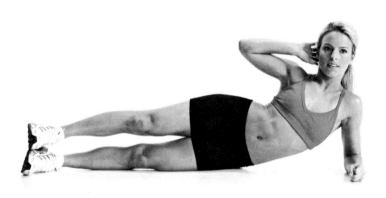

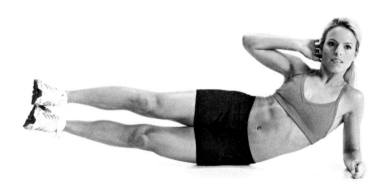

SIDE JACKKNIFE

Lie on your left hip, with your legs nearly straight and slightly raised off the floor. Also raise your torso off the floor, with your left forearm on the floor for balance. Hold your other hand behind your right ear, with your elbow pointed toward your feet. Lift your legs toward your torso while keeping your torso stationary. Pause to feel the contraction on the right side of your waist. Then slowly lower your legs and repeat. Finish the set on that side, then lie on your right hip and do the same number of repetitions.

10 repetitions each side [*Intermediate to advanced*]

Transverse Abdominis

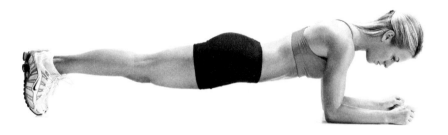

BRIDGE

Start to get in a Pushup position, but bend your elbows and rest your weight on your forearms instead of your hands. Your body should form a straight line from your shoulders to your ankles. Pull your abdominals in; imagine you're trying to move your belly button back to your spine. Hold for 20 seconds, breathing steadily. As you build endurance, you can do one 60-second set.

1 to 2 repetitions [*Beginner to intermediate*]

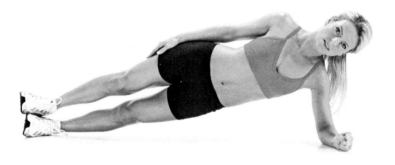

SIDE BRIDGE

Lie on your nondominant side. Support your weight with that forearm and the outside edge of that foot. Your body should form a straight line from head to ankles. Pull your abs in as far as you can and hold this position for 10 to 30 seconds, breathing steadily. Relax. If you can do 30 seconds, do one repetition. If not, try for any combination of reps that gets you up to 30 seconds. Repeat on your other side.

1 to 2 repetitions each side [*Beginner to intermediate*]

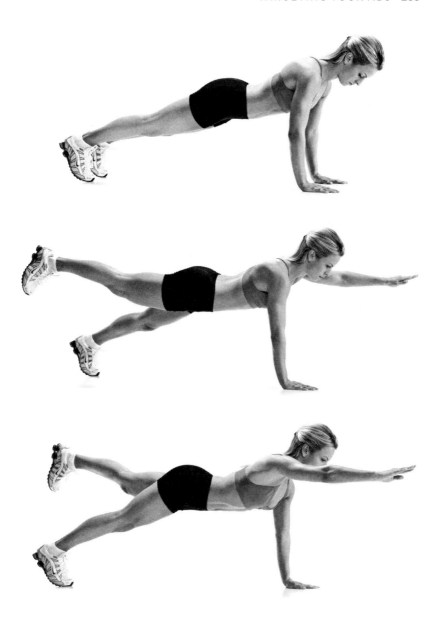

TWO-POINT BRIDGE

Get into the standard Pushup position. Lift your left arm and your right leg off the floor at the same time. Hold for 3 to 5 seconds. That's one repetition. Return to the starting position, then repeat, lifting your right arm and left leg this time.

6 to 10 repetitions each side [*Intermediate*]

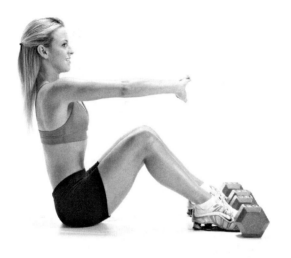

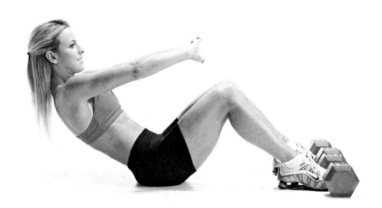

NEGATIVE CRUNCH

Sit on the floor with your knees bent and your feet flat on the floor and shoulder-width apart. Extend your arms with your fingers interlaced, palms facing your knees. Begin with your upper body at slightly less than a 90-degree angle to the floor. Lower your body toward the floor, curling your torso forward, rounding your lower back, and keeping your abs contracted. When your body reaches a 45-degree angle to the floor, return to the starting position. (Note: You may need to tuck your feet under a set of weights to help maintain balance throughout the exercise.)

10 repetitions [*Intermediate*]

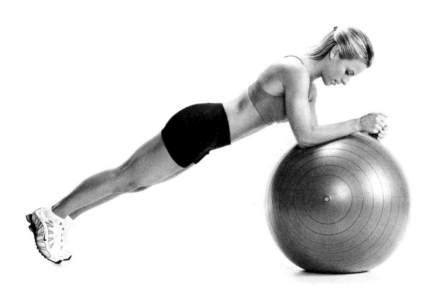

SWISS BALL BRIDGE

Rest your forearms on a Swiss ball and your toes on the floor, with your body in a straight line. Pull your stomach in, trying to bring your belly button to your spine. Hold for 20 seconds, breathing steadily. As you build endurance, you can do one 60-second set.

1 to 2 repetitions [*Intermediate to advanced*]

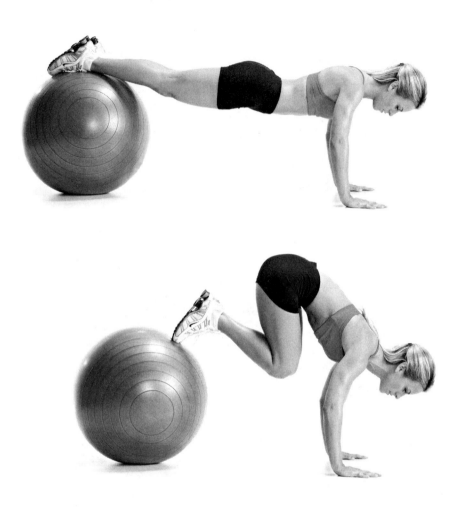

SWISS BALL PULL-INS

Get into the pushup position—your hands set slightly wider than and in line with your shoulders—but instead of placing your feet on the floor, rest your shins on a Swiss ball. With your arms straight and your back flat, your body should form a straight line from your shoulders to your ankles. Roll the ball toward your chest. Pause, then return the ball to the starting position by extending your legs and rolling the ball backward.

5 to 10 repetitions [*Intermediate to advanced*]

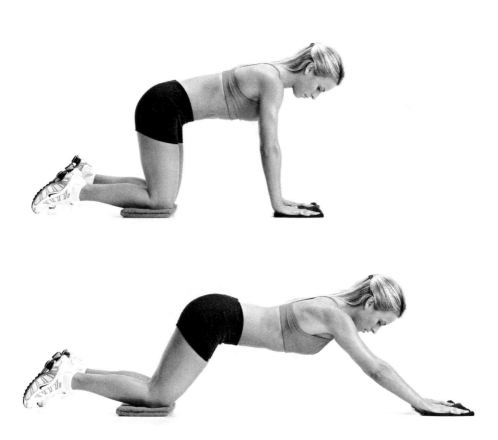

TOWEL ROLL

Kneel on a towel or mat on a tile or wooden floor. Put a towel on the floor in front of you, and place your hands on it. Slide the towel across the floor until your body is fully extended. Your body should look as if you're in a diving position. Slowly slide back up.

5 to 10 repetitions [*Advanced*]

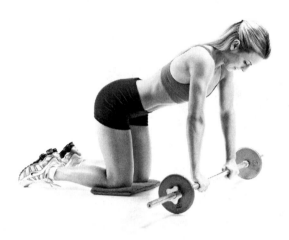

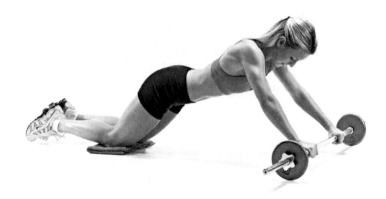

BARBELL ROLLOUT

Load a pair of 5-pound plates onto a barbell. Kneel on an exercise mat or towel, with your shoulders directly over the bar. Grab the bar with an overhand, shoulder-width grip. Start with your back in a slightly rounded position, allowing it to extend into a more neutral position as you execute the movement. Roll the bar out in front of you, holding your knees in place as your hips, torso, and arms go forward. Keeping your arms taut, advance as far as you can without arching your back or touching the floor with anything above your knees. Pause for a split second, then pull back to the starting position.

5 to 10 repetitions [*Advanced*]

Lower Back

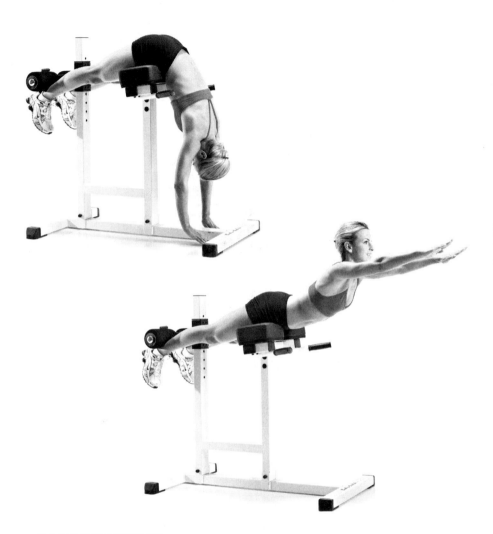

BACK EXTENSION

Position yourself in a back extension station and hook your feet under the leg anchor. Hold your arms straight out in front of you. Your body should form a straight line from your hands to your hips. Lower your torso, allowing your lower back to round, until it's just short of perpendicular to the floor. Raise your upper body until it's slightly above parallel to the floor. At this point, you should have a slight arch in your back, and your shoulder blades should be pulled together. Pause for a second, then repeat.

12 to 15 repetitions [*Beginner to intermediate*]

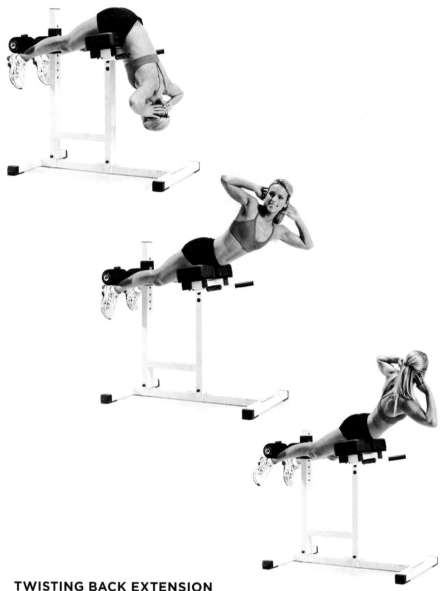

TWISTING BACK EXTENSION

Position yourself in a back extension station and hook your feet under the leg anchor. Place your fingers lightly behind or over your ears. Lower your upper body, allowing your lower back to round, until it's just short of perpendicular to the floor. Raise and twist your upper body until it's slightly above parallel to the floor and facing right. Pause, then lower your torso and repeat, this time twisting to the left.

12 to 15 repetitions [*Intermediate*]

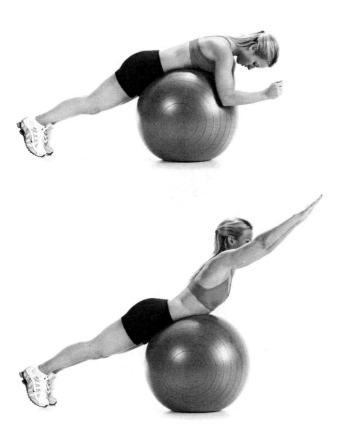

SWISS BALL SUPERMAN

Lie facedown over a Swiss ball so that your hips are pressed against the ball and your torso is rounded over it. Lift your upper arms so that they're parallel to your body, and bend your elbows 90 degrees so that your hands are pointing forward and your elbows are pointing back. Slowly extend your back until your chest is completely off the ball, extend your arms forward, and hold that position. Draw your arms back into position as you return your torso to the ball.

12 to 15 repetitions [*Intermediate*]

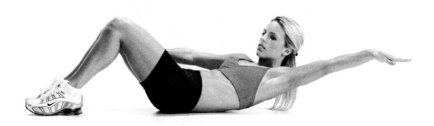

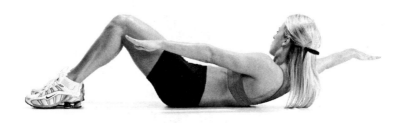

SWIMMER'S BACKSTROKE

Lie faceup on the floor, with your knees bent and feet flat. Flatten your lower back against the floor. Now do a crunch to flex your trunk forward and lift your shoulder blades as high off the floor as you possibly can. Keeping your chest high, perform a backstroke with one arm at a time, allowing your torso to twist toward the arm that's reaching back. Work up to 5 repetitions of 45 seconds each, alternating arms. The higher you lift your chest off the floor, the better the exercise will work. Add light dumbbells when this move becomes too easy.

1 to 5 repetitions [*Intermediate to advanced*]

12 Above-the-Belt Time-Savers!

LOOKING TO SHAVE even more time off your workout while shaving fat from your waistline? The following 12 moves of our 50-"six-pack" plan work several areas of your midsection simultaneously. Use any one of the following substitutions to cover two or three areas with one exercise, and you can reduce your workout plan to just a few exercises instead of five!

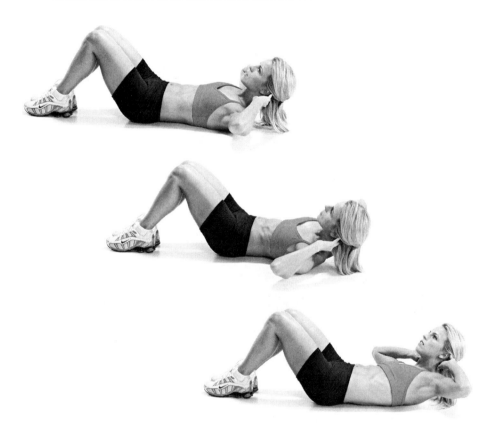

CRUNCH/SIDE BEND COMBO
Targets both the upper abs and obliques

Lie on your back, with your knees bent and your hands behind your ears. Curl up so that your shoulder blades are off the floor. Bend at the waist to the left, aiming your left armpit toward your right hip. Straighten, then bend to your right.

8 repetitions each side [*Beginner*]

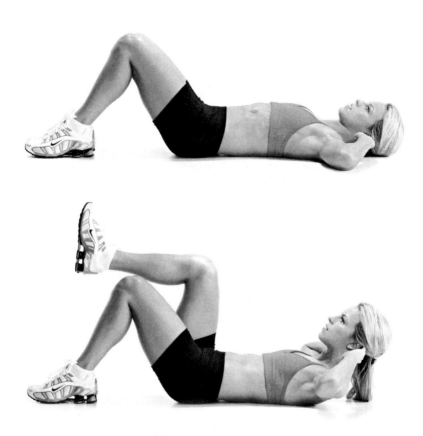

SINGLE-KNEE CRUNCH
Targets both the upper and lower abs

Lie on your back, with your knees bent so that your feet are flat on the floor. Touch your fingers to the sides of your head, with your elbows bent. Raise your head, shoulders, and butt off the floor as you simultaneously bring your right knee toward your chest. Lower your torso and leg back down, then repeat the exercise, this time drawing your left knee up instead as you crunch.

10 repetitions each side [Beginner to intermediate]

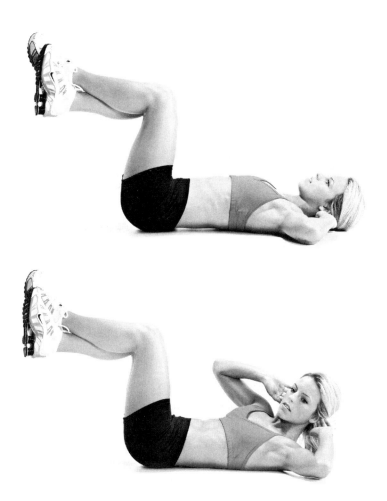

TWISTING CRUNCH

Targets both the upper abs and obliques

Lie on your back on the floor, with your hands cupped behind your ears and your
elbows out. Cross your ankles, with your knees slightly bent, and raise your legs
until your thighs are perpendicular to your body. Bring your right shoulder off the
floor as you cross your right elbow over to your left knee. Return to the starting
position and repeat, beginning with the left shoulder, crossing your left elbow
over to your right knee.

8 repetitions each side [*Beginner to intermediate*]

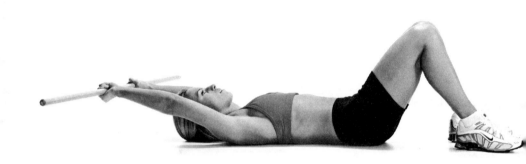

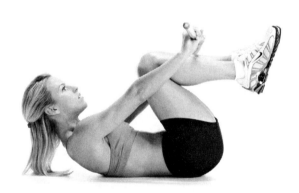

STICK CRUNCH
Targets both the upper and lower abs

Lie on your back, with your knees bent and your feet flat on the ground.
Hold a broomstick behind your head, with your arms extended and off
the ground. Crunch your torso up and draw your knees up so that the stick
extends past your knees. Pause, then return to the starting position.

12 repetitions [*Intermediate*]

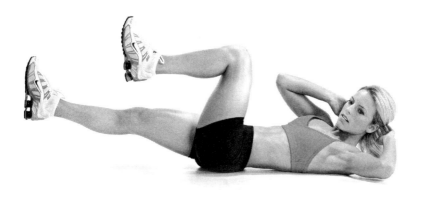

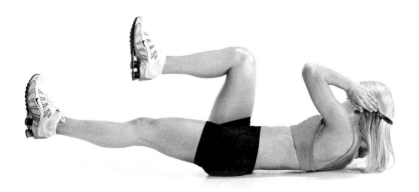

BICYCLE
Targets both the upper and lower abs

Lying on your back with your knees bent 90 degrees and your hands behind your ears, pump your legs back and forth, bicycle-style, as you rotate your torso from side to side by moving an armpit (not an elbow) toward the opposite knee.

20 repetitions [*Intermediate*]

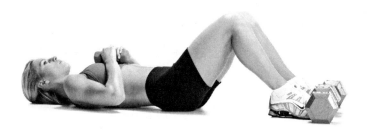

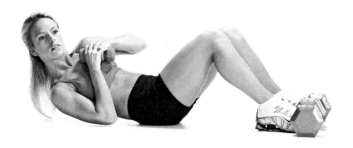

WEIGHTED ONE-SIDED CRUNCH

Targets both the upper abs and obliques

Lie with your knees bent and feet flat on the floor. Hold a dumbbell by your left shoulder with both hands. Curl your torso up and rotate to the right. Lower yourself, finish the set, then repeat, placing the dumbbell next to your right shoulder.

8 repetitions each side [*Intermediate*]

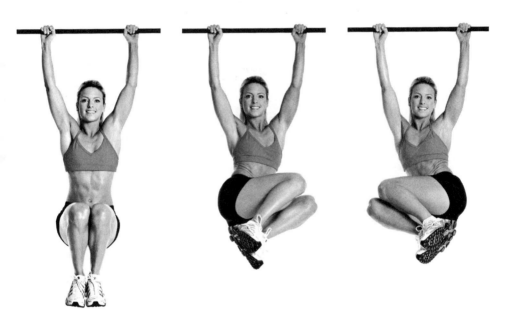

OBLIQUE HANGING LEG RAISE
Targets both the lower abs and obliques

Grasp a chinup bar with an overhand grip and hang from it at arm's length, with your knees bent. Keep your knees bent and lift your right hip toward your right armpit until your lower legs are nearly parallel to the floor. Pause, then return to the starting position, and lift your left hip toward your left armpit.

10 repetitions each side [*Intermediate*]

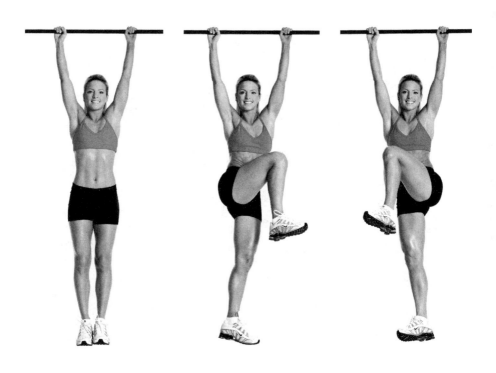

HANGING SINGLE-KNEE RAISE
Targets both the lower abs and obliques

Hang fully extended from a chinup bar, with your palms facing out and your hands a little farther than shoulder-width apart. Your feet should lightly touch the floor. Without swinging to pick up momentum, raise your right knee toward your left shoulder as far as you can, using your abs for power. Slightly thrust your pelvis forward to help, but don't rock. Hold for a second, then lower to the starting position. Repeat with your left leg, raising it toward your right shoulder.

8 to 12 repetitions each side [*Intermediate*]

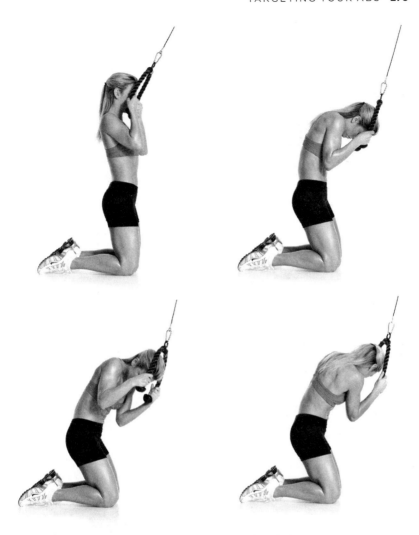

KNEELING THREE-WAY CABLE CRUNCH
Targets both the upper abs and obliques

Attach a rope to the handle of the high pulley. Kneel facing the pulley, and grab the ends of the rope, with your palms facing each other. Hold the rope along the sides of your face, with your elbows slightly bent. Bend forward at the waist, rounding your back and aiming your chest at your pelvis. Stop when you feel a contraction in your abdominal muscles. Return to the starting position, then repeat the movement, this time aiming your chest toward your right knee. Stop when you feel a contraction in your right obliques. Return, then repeat the movement to your left. That's 1 repetition.

8 repetitions [*Intermediate to advanced*]

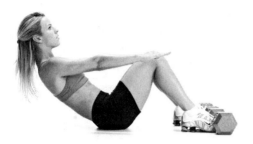

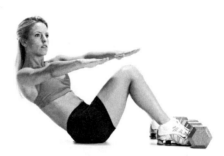

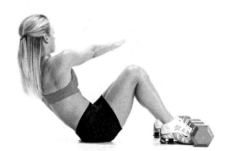

RUSSIAN TWIST

Targets both the upper abs and obliques

Sit on the floor, with your knees bent and your feet flat. Hold your arms straight out in front of your chest, with your palms facing down. Lean back so that your torso is at a 45-degree angle to the floor. Twist to the right as far as you can, pause, then reverse your movement and twist all the way back to the left as far as you can. As you get stronger, hold a light weight in your hands as you do the movement. (Note: You may need to tuck your feet under a set of weights to help maintain balance throughout the exercise.)

10 repetitions each side [*Intermediate to advanced*]

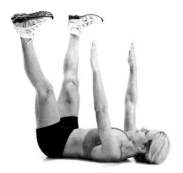

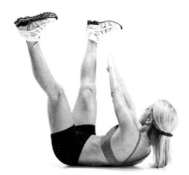

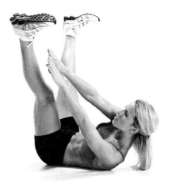

V-SPREAD TOE TOUCH

Targets both the upper abs and obliques

Lie flat on your back, with your legs straight up in a V position without locking your knees. Raise your arms toward the ceiling. Curl your shoulder blades up and reach toward your right foot with both hands. Hold for a second, concentrating on your abs, then lower to the starting position. Repeat, this time reaching for your left foot. Don't pause at the lower position.

12 to 15 repetitions [*Intermediate to advanced*]

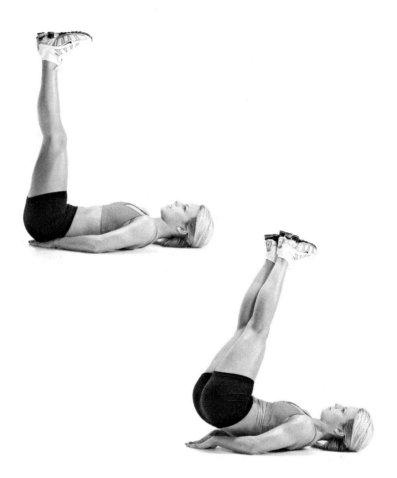

CORKSCREW
Targets both the lower abs and obliques
Lie on your back, with your legs raised directly over your hips; your knees should
be slightly bent. Place your hands with the palms down at your sides. Use your lower
abs to raise your hips off the floor and toward your rib cage, elevating your hips
straight up toward the ceiling. Simultaneously twist your hips to the left in a cork-
screw motion. Hold, then return to the starting position. Repeat, twisting to the right.

10 repetitions [*Intermediate to advanced*]

The No-Crunch Abs Workout

MAYBE YOU JUST can't stomach a crunch, or want to take a break from doing them. The remaning five moves will give you a tight stomach without doing a single crunch. This workout combines fat-burning cardio with moves that target your entire core rather than individual muscles. Do it as a circuit, one exercise immediately after the other.

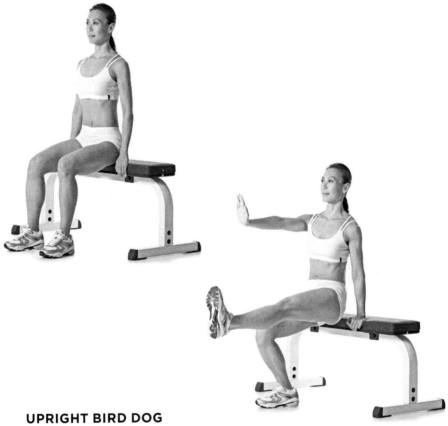

UPRIGHT BIRD DOG

Sit on the edge of your chair with your feet flat on the floor, resting your hands on the seat next to your hips. Keep your hips, knees, and ankles bent 90 degrees. Shift your weight forward off the seat so that all your weight rests on your hands and feet. Bracing your abs and keeping your torso stable, lift your left foot off the floor and your right arm straight in front of you. Hold for 10 seconds, then repeat the move with the opposite arm and leg. That's 1 rep.

10 repetitions [*Beginner*]

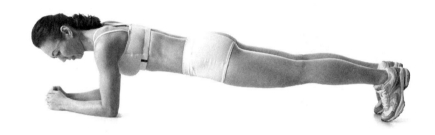

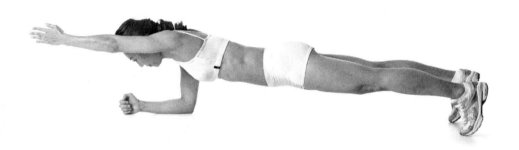

PLANK WITH ARM LIFT

Get into the plank position (toes and forearms on the floor, body lifted). Your body should form a straight line. Brace your abs and carefully shift your weight to your right forearm. Extend your left arm in front of you and hold for 3 to 10 seconds. Slowly bring your arm back in. Repeat with the right arm. That's 1 rep.

10 repetitions [*Intermediate to advanced*]

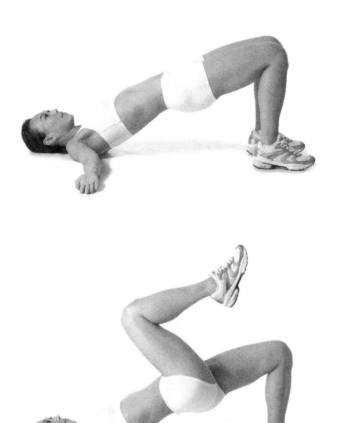

GLUTE BRIDGE MARCH

Lie on your back with your knees bent and your feet flat on the floor. Rest your arms on the floor, palms up, at shoulder level. Raise your hips so your body forms a straight line from your shoulders to your knees. Brace your abs and lift your right knee toward your chest. Hold for 2 counts, then lower your right foot. Repeat with the other leg. That's 1 rep.

10 repetitions [*Intermediate*]

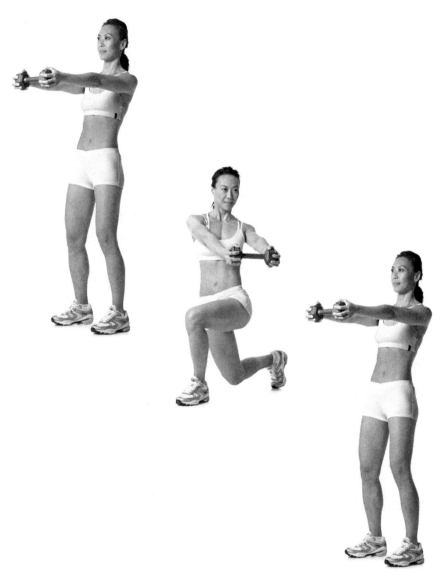

LUNGE WITH ROTATION

Grab a 5- to 15-pound dumbbell with both hands. Stand with your feet hip-width apart and your arms straight out. Take a big step forward with your left foot and, bracing your abs, twist your torso to the left as you bend your knees and lower your body until both of your legs form 90-degree angles. Keep your elbows straight but not locked. Twist back to center, push off your left foot, and stand back up. Repeat with the other leg. That's 1 rep.

10 repetitions [*Intermediate to advanced*]

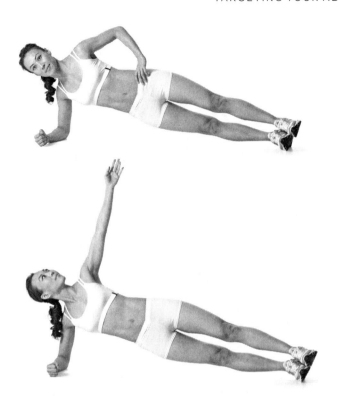

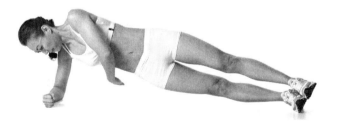

SIDE PLANK WITH ROTATION

Get into a side plank position supporting yourself with your right forearm. Brace your abs and reach your left hand toward the ceiling. Slowly tuck your left arm under your body and twist forward until your torso is almost parallel to the floor. Return to the side plank. After 10 reps, switch to your left side and do the reach up-and-under with your right arm.

10 repetitions [*Advanced*]

Special Bonus Section

LOOK HOT IN YOUR JEANS

Leg-Toning and Butt-Shaping Exercises for Your Abs Diet Workout

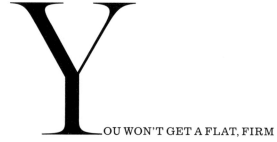

OU WON'T GET A FLAT, FIRM belly only by doing exercises that blast your midsection. You need to work your entire body to build lean muscle that will help you burn fat. The best fat burner of all: your leg muscles. You can chew up a lot of fat by adding some muscle to them. Added bonus: You'll tone and firm them at the same time. And what woman doesn't want a firmer, tighter, more shapely butt, thighs, and calves? Try some of the leg- and butt-specific exercises on the following pages. Use them as exercise substitutes or to add to your Abs Diet Circuit.

||||||||||||||||||||||||||||||||||||||||||||||||||||||||||||||||||||||||||||||||||||||||||||||||||||||||||||||||||||||||||||||||||||

Stretch It Out

If your hamstrings are tight, you may develop the habit of leaning backward to relieve the pressure. This tends to thrust your belly forward, making you look paunchy. Stretching your hamstrings and hips a few times a week will help: Lie down and bend your right knee to 90 degrees to stabilize your hips, and press the small of your back against the floor. Keeping your left knee as straight as possible, lift that leg off the floor with your hands clasped behind your knee so your foot points toward the ceiling. Hold for 30 seconds, then switch legs.

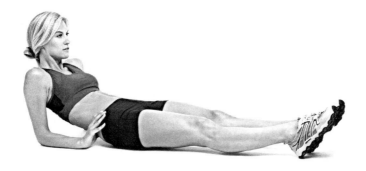

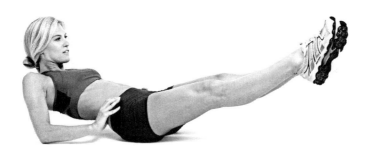

HALF-SEATED LEG CIRCLE

Sit on the floor with your legs fully extended, leaning back on your elbows, your fingers cupping the sides of your hips. Keeping your lower back pressed into the floor, engage your core and lift your legs about 45 degrees off the floor. Point your toes, press your thighs together, and trace 12 large clockwise circles, then 12 counterclockwise circles. Try to keep your pelvis still.

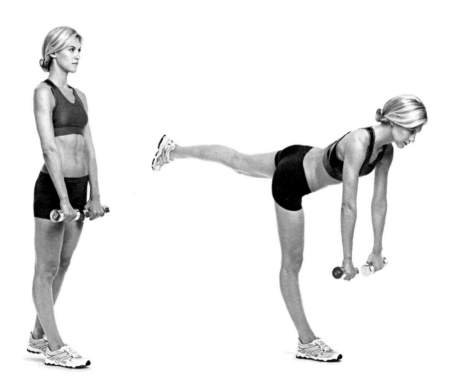

ALTERNATE-LEG DEAD LIFT

Hold a 5- to 15-pound dumbbell in each hand and stand on your right leg, lifting your left leg a few inches behind you. Keeping your back straight, lean forward from your hips until your body is almost parallel to the floor, the weights in line with your shoulders. Return to start. That's 1 rep. Do 12, then switch legs.

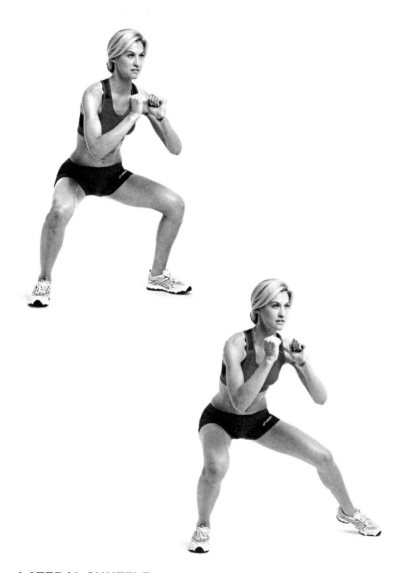

LATERAL SHUFFLE

Stand with your feet slightly wider than shoulder-width apart and turned out 45 degrees. Bend into a squat with your knees over your ankles. From that position, step to the left with your left foot, keeping your knees bent in the squat position. Take a step to the left with your right foot to return to start. Continue moving quickly sideways, taking 10 steps to the left and then 10 to the right.

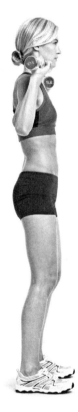
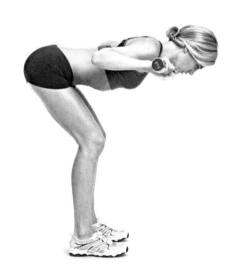

GOOD MORNING BEND

Stand with your feet shoulder-width apart and hold a pair of 5- to 15-pound dumb-bells at your shoulders, palms facing forward. Keeping your knees slightly bent and your torso straight, slowly bend from your hips until your upper body is parallel to the floor. Hold for 5 seconds and return to start. That's 1 rep; do 8 to 10.

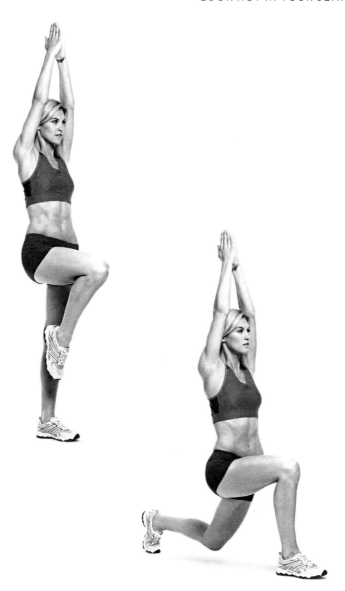

STABILITY LUNGE

Stand with your feet shoulder-width apart and your arms at your sides. Lift your right knee until your thigh is parallel to the floor and raise your arms overhead, palms facing in. Hold for 5 seconds, then slowly drop your right foot into a front lunge. Bring your left leg forward and return to standing. That's 1 rep. Do 10 to 12 on each leg, alternating sides. Tip: Make it harder by holding a dumbbell.

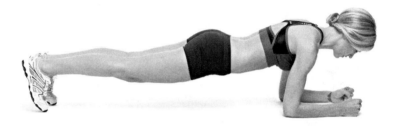

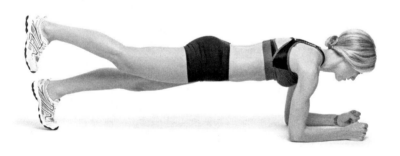

SINGLE-LEG PLANK

Get on the floor and prop yourself up with your toes flexed underneath you and
your elbows under your shoulders, shoulder blades back and down. Your body
should form a straight line. Brace your abs and lift your right leg up about 10 inches.
Balance your body weight on your forearms and the stabilizing leg. Hold for up to
60 seconds. Switch legs and repeat on the other side.

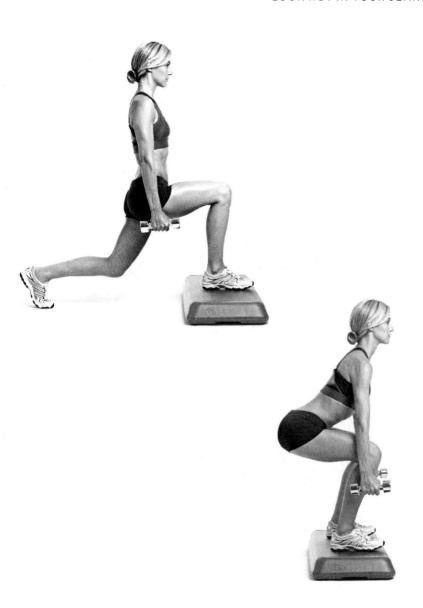

SKATER'S STEP-UP

Hold a pair of 5- to 15-pound dumbbells at hip level and stand facing a step with your right foot planted on the step. Leaning your chest forward slightly, lunge backward with your left leg, bending your right knee 90 degrees. From that position, bring your left foot up to meet the right on the step; squat and hold for 2 seconds. Stand and return to start. That's 1 rep. Repeat with the other leg; do 10 to 12 reps on each leg.

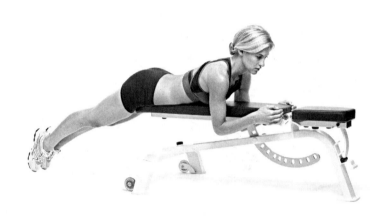

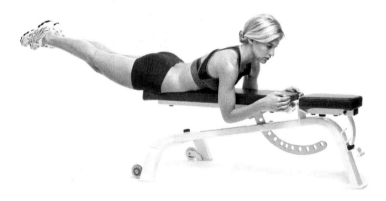

PRONE HIP EXTENSION

Lie facedown over a bench with your legs hanging off the edge. Engage your abs and glutes to lift both legs until your body forms a straight line. Hold for 5 seconds, then lower slowly. That's 1 rep; do 10 to 15.

Sculpt a Better Butt

FOR A SEXIER rear view, try these plyometrics-inspired moves that incorporate leaping, jumping, and skipping. These explosive movements shock your muscles so you'll see quick results. And their dynamic quality engages more muscle fibers than static resistance exercises do so you'll burn more calories. Try the following workout once a week. Start with 1 set of of each exercise, then add a set of each weekly until you reach 3 sets. Finish each workout with the inchworm and figure 4 stretches (pages 297, 298).

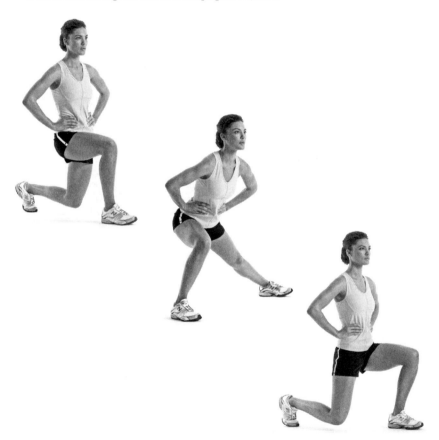

CLOCK LUNGE

With your hands on your hips, lunge forward with your right foot, sinking down until your right knee is bent 90 degrees. Return to standing. Take a big step to the right and lunge again. Step back to center. Lunge back with your right leg. That's 1 rep. Do 10, then repeat with your left leg.

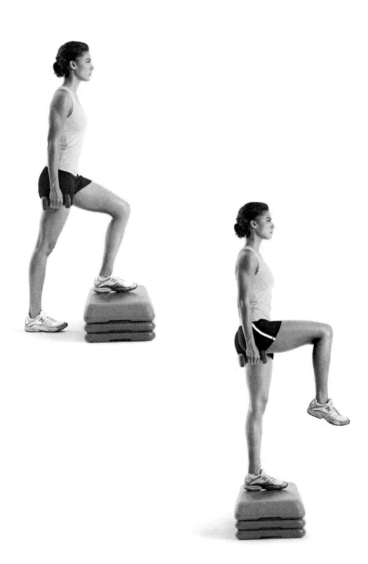

STEP-UP WITH KNEE RAISE

Place a 12- to 24-inch-high step in front of you. Step up with your left foot, bringing your right leg forward and up and bending your knee until your right thigh is parallel to the floor. Lower your right leg back to start, then the left. Repeat, this time with the right foot leading. That's 1 rep; do 10. (To make harder, hold 5- to 10-pound dumbbells.)

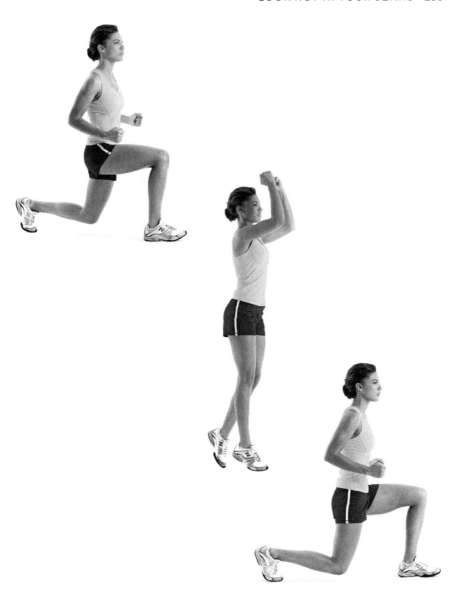

LUNGE JUMP

Stand with your feet together, elbows bent 90 degrees. Lunge forward with your right foot. Jump straight up as you thrust your arms forward, elbows still bent. Switch legs in midair, like a scissor, and land in a lunge with your left leg forward. Repeat, switching legs again. That's 1 rep; do 10.

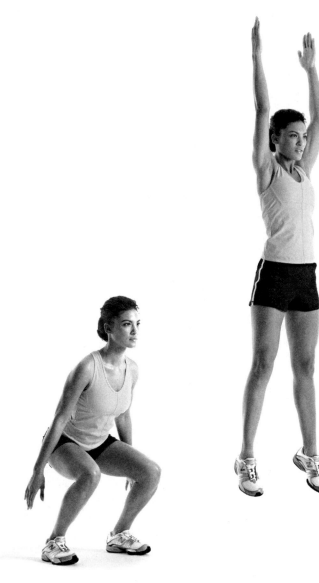

SQUAT JUMP

Stand with your feet shoulder-width apart, arms hanging at your sides. Squat down until your knees are bent about 90 degrees. Immediately swing your arms overhead and jump upward as high as you can. (Swinging your arms will give you momentum so you can catch more air.) As you land, gently bend your knees and sink back down into the squat position. That's 1 rep; do 10.

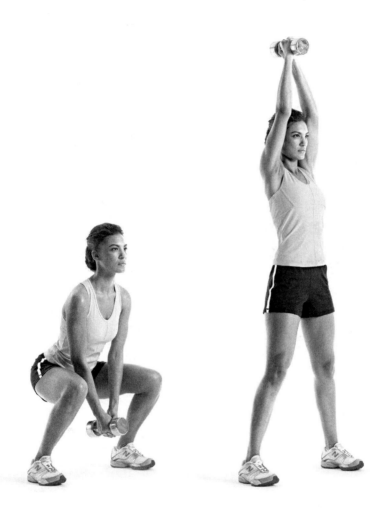

WOOD CHOPPER

Grab an 8- to 10-pound dumbbell with both hands and stand with your feet shoulder-width apart. Let the dumbbell hang naturally in front of your thighs. Squat down until your knees are bent about 90 degrees. Keeping your elbows slightly bent, brace your abs and press up to standing, swinging the dumbbell up until it's directly overhead. Lower the dumbbell back toward the floor. That's 1 rep; do 10.

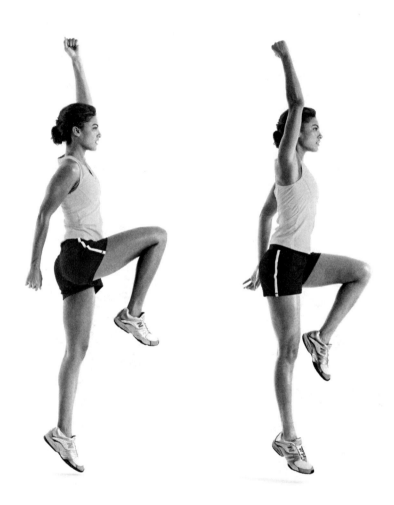

POWER SKIP

Leading with your right leg, skip as high as you possibly can by raising your right knee to hip height and simultaneously extending your left arm straight overhead. Your left leg should remain straight and your right elbow should be slightly bent at your side. Land on the ball of your left foot. Repeat the skipping motion with your opposite arm and leg. That's 1 rep; do 10.

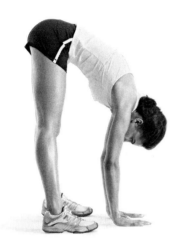

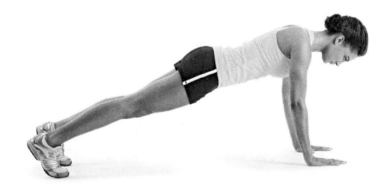

INCHWORM STRETCH

Standing with your feet hip-distance apart, slowly bend at the waist, keeping your legs as straight as possible, until your hands touch the floor about 8 to 12 inches from your feet. Walk your hands out to pushup position, then walk your feet in toward your hands. Work up to 2 sets of 8 reps.

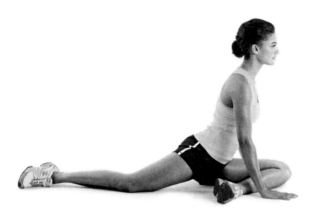

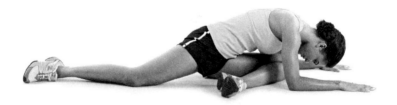

FIGURE 4 STRETCH

Starting out on all fours, cross your left leg under your body, so that you are almost resting on your left hip. Extend your right leg directly behind you. Lower your upper body over your left leg, placing your forearms on the ground in front of you. Hold for 30 seconds, then switch sides.

The One-Move Workout!

CRUNCHED FOR TIME? At the very least, you can do an exercise that works many of your major muscles at once. The move shown below works almost all of your big muscles simultaneously, especially the legs and butt, so you burn more calories per rep. It also strengthens your whole core, so you'll have better balance and stability and be less prone to lower-back injuries.

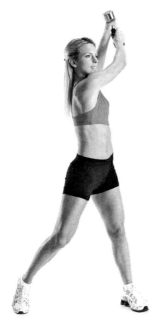 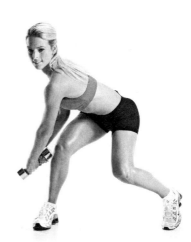

DIAGONAL CHOP

Hold a dumbbell with both hands in front of your body and raise it up over your head as you pivot on your right foot and rotate your body to the left, lifting the dumbbell up over your left shoulder. Lower your body and chop the dumbbell down toward your right foot, allowing your feet to pivot. You'll end up in a lunge position. Rotate back to the left, lifting your body and bringing the dumbbell back up. Repeat for 10 reps before switching sides. Add some variation with these three changes.

▶ **Go faster:** If you speed up your pace, it will force your core to work harder to stabilize your body as you squat, twist, and lift.

▶ **Extend your reach:** By reaching out more over your toe (and extending farther over your shoulder), you'll add more leverage to the exercise and increase your range of motion.

▶ **Get heavy:** Heavier weight equals heavier sweat.

Chapter 16

THE ABS DIET AND YOUR HORMONES

How the Program Can Work with Your Body's Natural Cycles

AY THE WORD HORMONES to a man and the only thing he thinks about is the next time he's going to indulge his. But say the word to a woman, and she understands the complexity, the nuances, and the power that her hormones have. They control moods, they control reproduction, and they can control whether you burn fat or store it.

Though they often seem to be unleashed like a pit bull in a butcher shop, hormones can be kept under control—if you know what to do. Research shows that there are many things you can do to keep your hormones functioning at normal levels, whether you're experiencing natural drops in estrogen that happen during the aging process or you're having trouble burning fat because of a thyroid hormone that's fritzing out like your aunt's 1973 TV set. These strategies will help you manage the fluctuating hormone levels you may be experiencing, all while adopting the Abs Diet as your new, fat-burning, body-changing lifestyle.

Beat PMS

Popping OTC medication isn't the only thing you can do to help alleviate the cramps, foul moods, and hunger that come with the fluctuating levels of estrogen and progesterone you experience before your period. Try these easy lifestyle changes that can ease some of the cyclical burden.

▶ Even more than you usually do on the Abs Diet, focus on eating protein and fiber to keep your blood sugar even, slow your rate of digestion, and resist the urge to overeat. The best foods include whole grains, fruits, and vegetables.

▶ A University of Massachusetts at Amherst study found that a high intake of calcium and vitamin D decreases the severity of PMS symptoms, plus it prevents PMS from initially developing. The study concluded that women who ate or drank about 1,200 milligrams of calcium and 400 IU of vitamin D daily had significantly lower risk of developing PMS. That's the equivalent of four servings a day of fat-free or low-fat milk, other low-fat dairy products like yogurt, or fortified orange juice.

▶ Have the perfect breakfast. It combines vitamin B6 with magnesium (both found in salmon and avocados), two nutrients that have been shown to relieve monthly mood swings. This magical meal also includes cheese, which helps replenish the vitamin D and calcium that your period can deplete. And it features fiber: A high-fiber diet has been shown to ease PMS symptoms by expelling excess estrogen. Best, it includes three powerfoods! Here's the secret recipe.

2 slices 100 percent whole-grain bread, toasted

1 tablespoon low-fat cream cheese

¼ avocado

1 ounce smoked salmon

Freshly ground pepper

Small handful of alfalfa sprouts or fresh spinach

On one slice of toast, spread the cheese and layer the avocado and fish. Top with the pepper, sprouts, and second slice of toast.

▶ You can cut down on period-related migraines and headaches associated with drops in estrogen levels by eliminating foods that tend to trigger them. The most common foods include aged cheeses, processed meats with nitrates, chocolate, excessive caffeine, alcohol (especially red wine), citrus foods, bananas, aspartame, and MSG. Exercise and meditation also seem to help reduce the risk of developing migraines, partly because they reduce stress (a migraine trigger).

▶ A yoga pose that opens up the pelvic area can relieve bloating and cramps. Try a pose called reclining bound angle. To do it, sit on the floor with a long pillow behind you, of which the bottom should touch your sacrum, and a folded blanket should cover the top. Lie back into the pillow, resting your head on the blanket. Put the soles of your feet together and let your knees and thighs fall to the sides. Stay in the pose for 5 to 10 minutes and breathe deeply.

▶ A recent study found that taking 200 IU of vitamin E twice daily 2 days before—and 3 days during—menstruation can ease cramps. Those in the study who took the vitamin E experienced fewer than 2 hours of cramps per cycle, down from 17 on average. And only 4 percent of the women needed a pain reliever for cramp relief. The theory is that vitamin E hinders the formation of prostaglandins, the hormone-like chemicals that cause uterine contractions. But take E only for those 5 prescribed days each month; high doses taken over years at a time have been linked to heart trouble.

▶ Ask your doctor about tweaking your birth control regimen. In a Yale study, oral contraceptives reduced PMS symptoms by 50 percent in half the participants using 24 hormone pills and four sugar pills.

▶ Acupressure may also help ease symptoms. Research suggests that acupressure stimulates bloodflow and releases endorphins—the body's natural painkillers. In one study, those who had acupressure had 72 percent less pain (the same as those who took ibuprofen), while those who had a false acupressure treatment (not performed on the correct spots) had a 58 percent decrease.

Manage Menopause

LIFE IS FULL of transitions. You start a new job or watch your kids go off to kindergarten or adjust to a new season of *Survivor*. When it comes to her health, every woman has to deal with at least one major—and natural—transition. From a purely scientific standpoint, menopause—which usually occurs between ages 40 and 55—is defined as the period of time when a woman's ovaries stop producing eggs and her body ceases production of two major hormones: estrogen and progesterone (perimenopause is the start of these hormonal changes).

The outward sign is that menstruation becomes less and less frequent until it stops altogether. But it's also defined by many other signs because of the symptoms associated with the changing hormonal levels. These symptoms occur as your body finds ways to rebel against the declining hormonal levels.

Like a good bouillabaisse, all women aren't made the same way—especially when it comes to how they respond to menopause. While some women have mild symptoms, others have very severe responses; the severity of symptoms is usually caused by how suddenly or slowly the ovaries slow hormone production. The most common symptoms—hot flashes, insomnia, mood swings, vaginal dryness, infections, and a loss of sex drive—can also be accompanied by longer-term changes that can lead to such things as bone loss and higher cholesterol levels. Because menopause is a normal and natural aging process, it's not something you try to treat or prevent the way you would heart disease or cancer. Instead, your goal is to lessen the severity of the symptoms associated with it. Fortunately, there are many things that you can do naturally to decrease both the severity of symptoms and the risk of other problems that stem from menopause.

Use the New Abs Diet to keep your weight down. In the Iowa Women's Health Study, researchers found that the risk of breast cancer for postmenopausal women was 44 percent higher for those who weighed more. The high-risk group had a body mass index of 29.5 or higher, while the low-risk group had a BMI of 23.5 or lower (page 62 showed you how to calculate your BMI). Related to that, another study found that maintaining weight helps reduce the risk of coronary problems in postmenopausal women. And that's important: A recent study of more than 60,000 women found that 17 percent had a moderate to high likelihood of having a silent heart attack (that's a heart attack with no noticeable symptoms). It's particularly important to keep an eye on your weight because this is an especially difficult time; one animal study showed that body weight can jump up 5 percent during menopause.

Bear fruit. Some fruits and vegetables contain phytoestrogens—elements that may trick the body into thinking it has higher levels of estrogen, which can help ease symptoms. Fruits with high phytoestrogens include plums, strawberries, apples, grapes, oranges, and raspberries. Vegetables include asparagus, cauliflower, broccoli, carrots, cucumbers, onions, and soybeans.

Go fish. Fish high in omega-3 fatty acids help add good cholesterol, which can help reduce the risk of heart attack (remember, it increases after menopause). You can also sub in flaxseed for additional omega-3s.

Embrace fat. Eating a small amount of dietary fat in one sitting can stimulate the gallbladder to empty, which helps prevent gallstones—which can be more common in menopause. Think almonds.

Go out shopping. And walk the aisles. A review of studies published in the journal *Sports Medicine* found that walking 30 minutes every day and one to three bouts of resistance training a week improved the health-related fitness of early postmenopausal women. The researchers determined the ranges by looking at the impact of various activities on bone mineral density, balance, insulin sensitivity, cholesterol, and body composition. Exercise may also help reduce menopausal symptoms by releasing endorphins—natural antidepressants that can help reduce incidences of insomnia, depression, mood swings, and headaches.

Huff. Though you may associate hot flashes with getting a glimpse of Usher's abs, they're more common in menopausal women for another reason. They occur because declining hormonal levels cause your internal thermostat to become unstable, making your body feel too hot. To cool down, blood vessels dilate and send a rush of blood to the surface of the skin—typically around your face, neck, and upper body. Your skin will get hot, you may sweat, and you may feel a prickly sensation during one of these flashes, which can last anywhere from 5 to 15 minutes. Hot flashes can cause all kinds of other symptoms, including insomnia and irritability. But you can decrease the effects of a hot flash with slow breathing exercises—go for slow, controlled breaths that last 10 seconds.

Keep a journal. As you enter perimenopause, you'll want to record information about your periods to note any irregularities in terms of flow or duration. But it's also smart to keep track of things that happen when you have hot flashes; you may find that you can identify the triggers—whether it's alcohol, spicy food, or hot weather—so you can figure out alternatives to avoid them.

Cohosh b'gosh. Black cohosh—an alternative remedy—has been shown in some studies to be effective at treating hot flashes.

Add water. As estrogen decreases in your body, you may experience vaginal dryness—increasing the chance of painful sex and decreasing the chance that you'll even want to make love. Water-based lubricants like Astroglide can help (avoid oil-based ones, which can actually dry out vaginal tissue).

Thyroid Hormone: The Metabolism-Busting Hormone

As you've probably figured out by now, there's a lot that goes into how your metabolism works—through what you eat and how you move. But eating sufficient protein and choosing a walk at lunch over Popeye's aren't the only things that control your metabolic rate. Your genetics plays a large part, too. As much as you can control your metabolism through your foods and exercise, you're not the sole controller of your metabolic odometer. Think of your metabolism as a little bit like an electric mixer: You have a very fast speed, a very slow speed, and lots of little speeds in between. That rate of mixing—or in your case, the rate at which you burn calories—varies a lot depending on how you control it. But your body also can short out—causing your calorie-mixer to go haywire or short out altogether. In a lot of ways, that controller comes in the form of your thyroid gland—a hormone-producing gland located in the front of your neck.

Your thyroid gland is like the new puppy of your body; it gets blamed for everything that can go wrong. Your thyroid gland doesn't just regulate metabolism; it also controls things like body temperature. But if something inside your body is causing your thyroid to malfunction, it throws off all of the systems it controls. That's where hyper- and hypothyroidism can affect your metabolism and how quickly or slowly you burn calories. Hypothyroidism is a condition in which the gland fails to produce enough thyroid hormone, meaning that your metabolism can grind to a crawl and lead to weight gain or at least make it very difficult to lose weight. Hyperthyroidism is the exact opposite. It's a condition where the gland overproduces thyroid hormone, so it increases metabolism to a point where you lose weight too fast (yes, there is such a thing). The added trouble is that thyroid hormone is also linked to the pituitary gland—meaning that any kind of problems in the production of thyroid hormone can also have an effect on brain functions that involve the pituitary. That's why thyroid troubles are often difficult to diagnose. Symptoms of hypothyroidism can come in the form of slow speech, abnormal menstrual periods, muscle pain, joint stiffness, drowsiness, swelling, and a host of others, while hyperthyroidism is marked by such things as rapid weight loss, intolerance to heat, restlessness, fatigue, sleeping trouble, and other symptoms.

It's also important to understand that your weight isn't the only thing your thyroid gland can mess up. One study showed that hypothyroidism increased the odds of heart disease by 70 percent and more than doubled the odds of a heart attack. That's why it's especially essential to have regular blood tests that can measure your levels of thyroid hormone. If the doctors determine your hormonal levels are off, they can prescribe medications to help put hormone levels back at a normal range.

Chapter 17

THE ABS DIET FOR MOMS

Using the Plan to Prepare for the Baby—
And Lose the Baby Weight

I T'S TRUE: SOME PEOPLE carry basketball-size bellies because of Death by Chocolate desserts and too many nosedives into the cheese fondue. But others carry big bellies because they're performing the single most important job in the world—carrying a child. Now, just because having a baby turns flat stomachs into bulbous ones doesn't mean that you should abandon a healthy eating and exercise lifestyle. In fact, it's even more important to maintain healthy habits before, during, and after pregnancy for your health and shape and that of your child. Just consider this study: Swedish researchers analyzed the weight of 563 women before, during, and 15 years after their pregnancies. They found that those who gained more than 35 pounds while expecting were $2^1/_2$ times more likely to keep the weight after birth. You want to shoot for a gain of between 25 and 35 pounds (that's the healthy range outlined by the American College of Obstetricians and Gynecologists). And studies show that being overweight while carrying a baby increases your risk of pregnancy-related problems such as gestational diabetes, preeclampsia, and Caesarean delivery.

Now, just because you'll lose your visible abs once you become pregnant doesn't mean the Abs Diet has to disappear as well. It's always vital for pregnant women to consult their doctors about any eating and exercise programs, but these are strategies for how the Abs Diet can be built for two.

Before Getting Pregnant . . .

DROP YOUR WEIGHT. Being overweight or obese raises your risk of gestational diabetes and therefore your child's risk of heart problems and birth defects. Gestational diabetes is also linked to abnormally large babies and difficult labor. Getting to a healthy weight is also important if you're considering in vitro fertilization (IVF). If you're 30 percent above your ideal weight while undergoing IVF, your odds of having a successful pregnancy are low. In one study, obese women were 32 percent less likely to get pregnant than were women with healthy weights. Researchers suspect that losing just 5 percent of body weight can improve odds—all the more reason to commit to the Abs Diet.

Watch the carbs. Refined carbs such as soda, cookies, fruit drinks, pretzels, and white bread may increase your baby's risk of birth defects. In a March of Dimes study, those who ate the largest amounts of refined carbohydrates during the 3 months before conception doubled the threat to their babies, compared with women who ate the least. Researchers suspect that starchy or sugary foods raise a woman's blood glucose, which can lead to cell damage and deplete the fetus of a chemical messenger between cells. The fix: powerfoods like whole grains, beans, and fruits and vegetables.

Exercise hard. A powerful incentive to do your high-intensity intervals: Researchers at the University of Washington who surveyed 688 mothers found that those who performed the most vigorous exercise during the year before pregnancy were 81 percent less likely to develop gestational diabetes than those who were sedentary, while moderate exercisers had a 59 percent lower risk.

Take folic acid. Take 400 micrograms of folic acid to help prevent birth defects, unless your multivitamin covers that amount. Be careful, though—the Food and Nutrition Board sets the safe upper limit for the nutrient at 1,000 micrograms. Good dietary sources include leafy green vegetables like spinach and fortified cereals.

Get a blood sugar check. It needs to be at a healthy level for 3 to 6 months before conception because unhealthy levels lead to increased risk of birth defects. If you have a family history of diabetes or are overweight, you're more at risk.

During Pregnancy . . .

KEEP WORKING OUT. Now, I'm not saying you should be signing up for marathons or trying your first 5-day adventure race, but exercising is important throughout pregnancy to maintain control of your weight as well as your tone. If you're a runner, you can keep running early in your pregnancy, but swimming is thought to be the safest cardiovascular exercise because it helps maintain body tone without stressing the joints. The one significant change you'll want to make to the Abs Diet program is to eliminate the interval workout. Doctors recommend that you keep your heart rate away from high-intensity levels. They recommend levels at which you can exercise and hold conversations at the same time—to ensure you don't overdo it. New research shows that physical activity can also make you less likely to deliver early.

Follow the Abs Diet Power 12. Though you need only 300 or so extra calories daily during the second and third trimesters, you need more of the food's nutrients to pass along. The recommended daily diet includes two to three servings of calcium-rich foods, three to five servings of vegetables, two to four of fruit, six to 11 of whole grains, and two to three of lean meats and other protein sources. (More below on specific nutrients.) Hmmm, by my count, that's the D, S, R, W, and T of ABS DIET POWER. Experts also recommend taking a multivitamin to ensure you're getting 400 micrograms of folic acid and calcium—the folic acid to protect against birth defects and the calcium to ensure you're getting enough to protect your bones. (The baby can take calcium away from your bones, leaving you at greater risk of osteoporosis.) Some specific recommendations:

▶ **Calcium:** Make sure you get at least 1,000 milligrams of calcium a day, about 200 milligrams more than before you were pregnant. An 8-ounce glass of milk has about 300 milligrams. Your doctor may prescribe or recommend a particular supplement; if not, Citracal is a reputable choice.

▶ **Iron:** The National Academy of Sciences suggests you get 27 milligrams of iron daily—9 more than before you were pregnant. This will likely require a supplement because a serving of beef—one of the best iron sources—contains only 3.5 milligrams.

▶ **Protein:** During pregnancy you'll need about 70 grams of protein a day. That's 20 more than usual. An additional ounce of cheese or serving of meat is enough.

Stick to six. Just because you're eating for two doesn't mean you can eat around the clock. If you get your six well-balanced meals, you'll be getting enough calories and nutrients for both of you. One interesting side note about what your baby needs: A study in the *British Medical Journal* reported on an experiment done on the dietary intake of 244 pregnant women in Boston. According to the researchers, pregnant women carrying males have a 10 percent higher energy intake than those carrying females. The male embryos ate 8 percent more protein, 9 percent more carbohydrates, 11 percent more animal fats, and 15 percent more vegetable fats. (See, even at an early age, we're trying to swipe stuff off your plate.) Researchers aren't sure why, but they speculate it could be caused by increased testosterone.

Now, if you're craving 16 meals a day instead of six, your best option is to try to combat cravings with handy, healthy snacks. Low-fat yogurt, low-fat cheese cubes, and baby carrots can help fend off some cravings, while dried

||||||||||||||||||||||||||||||||||||||||||||||||||||||||||||||||||||||||||||||||||||||||

The Mother of All Statistics

The average woman puts on 30 pounds while pregnant. Where it all goes:

▶ **Baby:** 7.5

▶ **Placenta:** 1.5

▶ **Amniotic fluid:** 2

▶ **Uterus:** 2

▶ **Breasts:** 2

▶ **Bodily fluids:** 4

▶ **Maternal stores of fat, protein, and other nutrients:** 7

▶ **Body parts, besides the belly, that temporarily increase by one full size:** bust and feet

▶ **Excluding the baby's weight, pounds lost immediately after delivery:** 11

fruit like apricots and raisins can help with a sweet pang. One really good option: Make small bags of homemade trail mix with nuts, granola, and a few pieces of dark chocolate. They'll help satisfy your sweet, salty, and crunchy cravings while also helping fill you up so you're less likely to gorge before your next meal. And if you're longing to down a tub of ice cream, you can satisfy the sweet tooth by having a cup of reduced-fat hot chocolate; it satisfies your chocolate urge, but its taste is lasting and the effect is satisfying because it takes a little longer to get through than, say, a candy bar.

Stay focused on fiber. University of Washington research shows that eating 21 grams of fiber a day lowers the risk of preeclampsia (the dangerous blood pressure condition) by about 70 percent, compared with eating less than 12 grams a day. Researchers attribute it to fiber's ability to lower blood pressure and cholesterol. You'll reach that mark by eating 2 cups of fruit, 2½ cups of vegetables, and three servings of whole grains.

Adjust your position. If you do yoga poses (as in Chapter 18), you should make slight adjustments to avoid putting your body in uncomfortable positions. Pass on postures that require you to contract or twist your abs, to avoid undue strain to the area, as well as poses that require you to lie on your belly. For standing poses, you might need to widen your stance to give your belly a little more room.

Consider ginger for nausea. Studies show that ginger is effective for relieving nausea and vomiting during pregnancy. Other studies show that ginger is as effective as vitamin B6 for effectively reducing severe nausea.

After You Give Birth . . .

GO BACK TO your abs workout after doctor's clearance. After you give birth, you may think your belly has reached the point of no return. But there are plenty of women who are able to regain their shape after pregnancy. It just takes a little longer. See, pregnancy stretches and weakens your abdominal muscles (C-sections weaken them even more). And it's not uncommon for some of the connective tissue around those abdominal muscles to take a year or more to return to its original strength. Ab exercises in any form work the muscles around your core to tighten and firm the entire area, and experts recommend exercises like Pilates and crunches to speed up the process. (You should always talk to your doctor about when it's safe for you to resume your workouts after childbirth.)

To start back slowly, try this exercise, which you can do while driving, sitting on the couch, or at your desk. Keeping your back supported, inhale and let your abdomen expand outward. Now exhale, drawing your abdominal muscles in, trying to bring your belly button toward your spine. Hold for a count of 30 (keep breathing). Then squeeze 10 times, pulling your belly button toward your spine with each contraction. Do it three times a day. By the way, your skin will go through similar changes as your muscles. But loose skin around the belly isn't a permanent problem. Skin is like an elastic band. When you stretch it, it'll eventually go back into shape. Tightening up post-pregnancy skin takes some time, but with those same ab-strengthening exercises, it can return to prepregnancy firmness. For a complete postpartum workout, see page 314.

Join a support group. New moms who attended 12 weekly diet and exercise education sessions lost an average of 16 pounds after a year, while those who attended a single educational session lost only 3 pounds, according to a Saint Louis University study. Check with your local hospital or community center to see if they have a postpartum weight loss class.

Have your thyroid checked. Up to 10 percent of all women suffer from postpartum thyroiditis, or a decline in thyroid levels after giving birth. That may mean your metabolism will slow down and you'll hold on to weight. Ask your doctor for a thyroid test if you are gaining weight, are really tired, or have joint and muscle aches. The right medications will put your metabolism back on track.

Breastfeed if possible. Yes, nursing is one of nature's greatest forms of exercise—it burns up to 500 calories a day. And a Cornell study shows that because of that calorie burn, women who breastfed for a year after giving birth were 2.6 pounds lighter than women who didn't. It also has weight-related benefits to your child. German research found that the longer a person was breastfed during infancy, the lower that person's risk of being overweight later in life. And the rates decreased for every month that the person was breastfed—with odds of being overweight being 32 percent lower for those who were breastfed more than 9 months, compared with those who were breastfed for less than a month.

But don't rely on breastfeeding to do all the work. While it's true that nursing burns calories, the results are not the same for everyone. In fact, 20 percent of nursing moms don't lose weight. Here are some specific things to watch out for while you're nursing.

▶ To avoid a drop in your milk volume, consume at least 1,800 calories a day. Just ditch foods that don't deliver nutritionally. Avoid calorie cutting for the first month after giving birth.

▶ Nursing moms need 1,000 milligrams of calcium and at least 200 IU of vitamin D every day from food and supplements to keep their bones healthy.

▶ Eat at least three servings of low-fat dairy and five servings of fruits and vegetables daily to avoid losing out on key nutrients. Note that some babies are allergic to the proteins in the cow's milk that their mothers consume. Most will lose the allergy symptoms (such as green stools or eczema) when their mothers eliminate dairy products. If this is your situation, you should consult your ob-gyn on the best way to ensure you're getting enough calcium.

Be patient. Getting your body back into shape after pregnancy is surely a postpartum stressor, but Johns Hopkins researchers say that most mothers get back their prepregnancy fitness levels just a few months after delivery. The researchers found that, no matter their fitness levels or BMIs, moms returned to their prepregnancy size within 27 weeks. Though their activities may have changed, their amount of activity stayed the same (less kickboxing, more walking with jog strollers).

The Postpartum Workout

As I SAID, when you want to resume your workouts after childbirth, you need to ask your doctor about when you can start back up, how much you can do, and what intensity is best. Most likely, she'll tell you to work your way back in slowly—heck, you've just been through nature's most intense workout ever. To ease back into your Abs Diet workouts, start with a little resistance exercise without using much weight at all. This workout will hit all of your major body parts without too much strain, and it will also serve as the signal to your body that you're ready to get back into action.

The Postpartum Workout

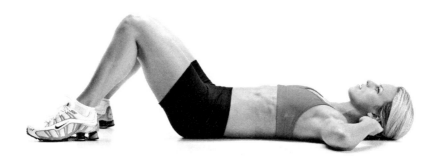

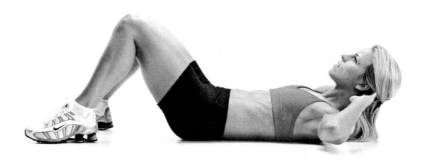

TRADITIONAL CRUNCH

Lie on your back with your knees bent and your hands behind your ears.
Slowly crunch up, bringing your shoulder blades off the ground. Hold this
position for 3 seconds, then return to the starting position. Do 10 repetitions.
Each week, increase by one the number of crunches you perform and the
number of seconds you hold each crunch.

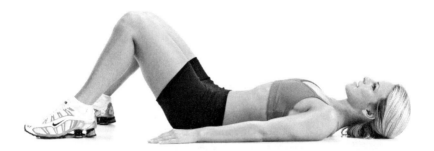

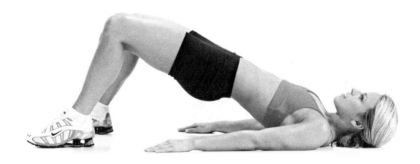

PELVIC TILT

Lie on your back with your knees bent and your feet flat on the floor. Inhale as you raise your buttocks and contract your abs. Hold for 5 seconds, then slowly lower, feeling each vertebra make contact with the floor. Repeat 10 times, increasing by two per week.

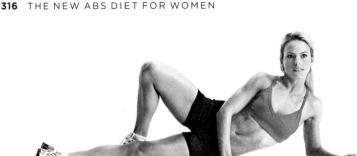

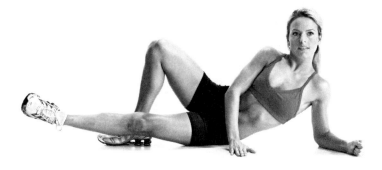

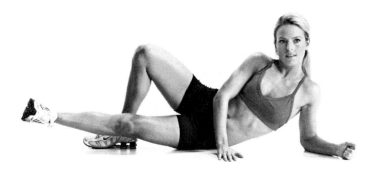

INNER THIGH LIFT

Lie on your left side, supporting yourself on your left elbow. Position your right hand in front of your body. Bend your right knee and position your right foot behind your left knee. Raise your left leg as high as you can, keeping your toes pointed. Slowly lower your leg. Repeat the motion, this time flexing your foot forward. Do the exercise 10 times, alternating between pointed toes and flexed foot (five times each). Then switch sides. Increase the number of repetitions you do by 2 each week.

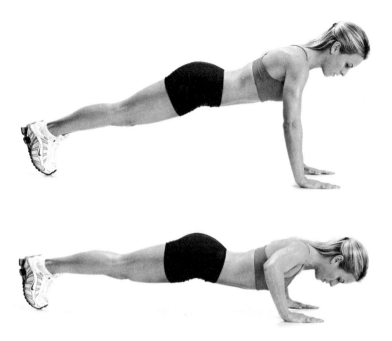

PUSHUP

Get in a pushup position with your hands about shoulder-width apart. Bend at the elbows while keeping your back straight, until your chin almost touches the floor, then push back up.

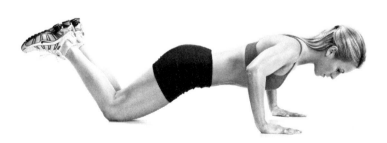

If this is too difficult, try it with your knees bent. Inhale as you raise your upper body, keeping your knees on the floor. Exhale as you lower your body. Do 10 repetitions, increasing the number of reps by 2 per week.

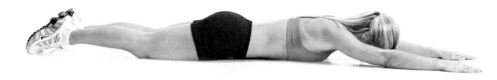

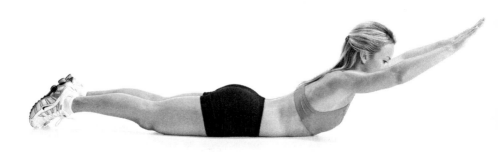

SUPERMOM

Lie flat on the floor with your legs straight and arms extended in front of you.
Without moving your legs, slowly lift your torso up off the floor as high as you
comfortably can, like Supermom flying off to comfort her crying baby. Pause, then
lower yourself back to the floor. Do 10 repetitions, increasing the number of reps
by 2 per week.

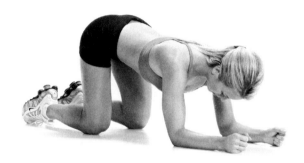

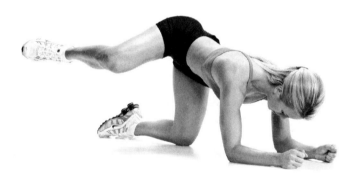

FIRE HYDRANT

Kneel with your hands, forearms, and elbows on the floor. Inhale and raise your right
leg out to the side, keeping your knee bent, until your thigh is parallel with the floor.
Exhale as you return to the starting position. Do 10 repetitions, then switch sides.
Increase the number of repetitions by 2 per week.

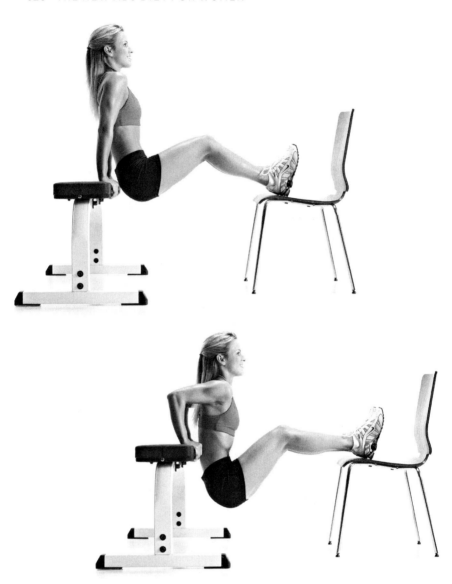

BENCH DIP

Stand with your back to a bench or chair and place your hands on the edge, fingers
pointing toward your lower back. Place your feet on a chair a few feet in front of
you. Keeping your hands in place, slowly step forward until your legs are extended
in front of you, knees slightly bent. Your arms should be straight, elbows unlocked,
supporting your weight. Slowly bend your arms to lower yourself as far as you can
and bring your butt as close to the floor as possible. Press yourself back up to the
starting position. Do 10 repetitions, increasing the number of reps by 2 per week.

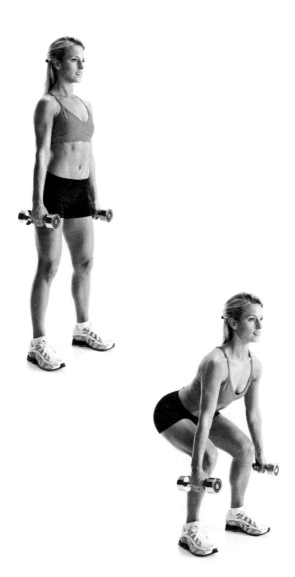

SQUAT

Holding a dumbbell in each hand, stand with your feet shoulder-width apart, and keep your knees slightly bent, back straight, arms at your sides, and eyes focused straight ahead. Slowly lower your body as if you were sitting back into a chair, keeping your back in its natural alignment and your lower legs nearly perpendicular to the floor. When your thighs are parallel to the floor, pause, then return to the starting position. Do 10 repetitions, increasing the number of reps by 2 per week.

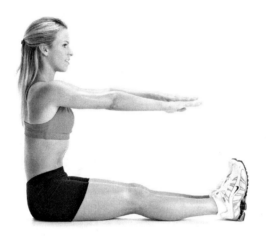

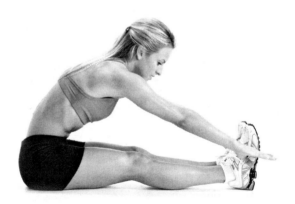

FORWARD STRETCH

Sit on the floor with your legs and arms stretched out in front of you. Exhale as you reach for your ankles or calves, bending your torso forward and leaning over your thighs. Hold for 10 to 15 seconds, then inhale as you return to an upright position. Repeat three times. Work up to 20 to 30 seconds per stretch and 5 repetitions.

Chapter 18

THE STRESS-BUSTING WORKOUT

A Program That Can Give You the Fit Body—
And Calm Mind—You Want

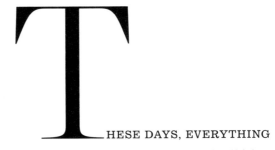HESE DAYS, EVERYTHING
is judged by how fast it can be. Fast food. Speed dating. Olympic athletes.
Internet connections. We're a society that's moving faster than autobahn
traffic—no speed limits, just cover as much ground as you can as fast as
you can. With all that we have to do, all the people we have to take care of, and
all the responsibilities we have, we're always on the move—trying to squeeze
every second with work, family, and, if we're lucky, a little bit of fun. What's that
mean? That our brains are packed like a 5 o'clock subway, and sometimes
we just crave the one thing that we can't get—the opportunity to step back.

And.

Slow.

Down.

Hey, I know you always have a lot on your plate (and it better be two or
three powerfoods!), but I also know the value of taking time for yourself to relax
and recharge. One of the best ways you can slow your mind is through classes
like yoga and Pilates. Softer and slower in pace, they can help relieve stress
and, when done to supplement your Abs Diet Workout, still give you a chal-

lenging enough workout throughout the week to add calorie burn and muscle tone. More and more evidence is showing the value of these kinds of workouts, no matter where you do them. For one, researchers at Jefferson Medical College took blood samples from yoga novices during a week when they took a 50-minute class. The results: Their levels of cortisol (the stress hormone) dropped immediately—even as soon as the first day of class.

And there's also evidence that yoga isn't just a spa sport anymore. In a University of Pittsburgh study, researchers put 59 obese, inactive women on a low-fat diet. Everyone walked for 40 minutes a day 5 days a week, but a third of the women did additional strength training, and another third added a yoga routine 3 days a week. After 4 months, the yogis dropped an average of 27 pounds—7 more than the walking-only group. (The strength group lost 23.)

In this chapter, I'll outline a few moves that you can use to supplement your strength-training, interval, and ab workouts. Do yoga moves one to three times a week—to clear your mind and stretch and work your muscles. As you get advanced with yoga moves, you can even choose a more vigorous style of yoga, like the vinyasa on page 337 or the Iron Yoga on page 343.

You can do moves at the end of a workout or as a separate session on your off days. For starters, try all of the poses once to see how they stretch your muscles, and then mix and match the poses for your workouts. During each session, aim to do four to six poses two or three times—holding each stretch for two full breaths (meaning that you inhale and exhale very slowly).

After the yoga poses, I've also included a section detailing some Pilates moves—moves that specifically work your core and will help build abdominal strength. You can substitute some of these Pilates moves, which start on page 349, for your ab workout.

||||||||||||||||||||||||||||||||||||||||||||||||||||||||||||||||||||||||||||||||||||||||||||||||||||||||

Walk This Way

Don't want to bring your yoga mat into your office cafeteria? Then walk it off. New research shows that you don't have to break a sweat to get mood-enhancing benefits from exercise. A brisk walk increases your heart rate, thus increasing bloodflow to your brain. That triggers the release of serotonin, the feel-good hormone that helps you feel energized and alert—not tense and stressed.

Yoga Poses

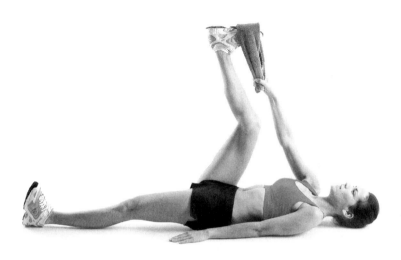

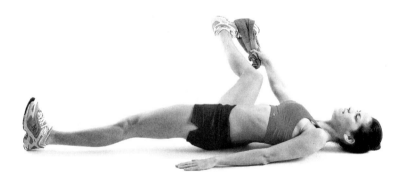

LYING DOWN LEG RAISE

Lie on your back and raise your right leg. Hold your right big toe with the first two fingers of your right hand (or hold a towel looped around your foot) and lower your leg smoothly toward your right shoulder. Go as far as you can and hold. Gently release and repeat with your left leg and hand.

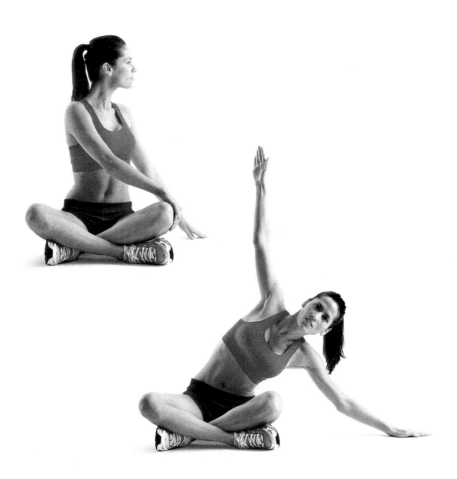

SPINAL STRETCH

Sitting cross-legged, press your butt bones into the floor and lengthen your spine, reaching up with the crown of your head. You can sit on a firm pillow or folded blankets if that's more comfortable. Place your right hand on your left knee, inhale and lengthen your spine, then exhale and twist to the left. Breathe, return to the center, switch sides, and repeat. Slide your left hand onto the floor and extend your right arm overhead. Inhale and reach your fingers up toward the ceiling, then exhale and reach to the left, stretching your right side. Breathe, switch sides, and repeat, reaching to the right.

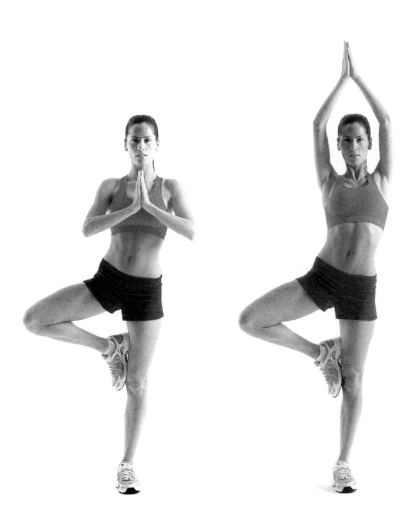

TREE

Stand with your feet rooted firmly to the floor. Keeping your left leg strong, bend your right leg and set your foot against the inside of your left thigh. Place your palms together in a prayer pose and extend your arms straight up to the ceiling. Hold, then switch legs.

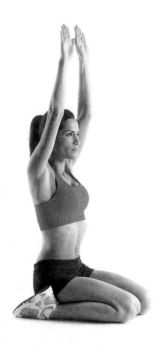

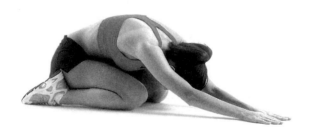

FORWARD HERO

Sit on your heels, then slide your heels out to the side so your butt is touching the floor. Sit upright, inhale, and raise both arms, bringing your elbows by your ears. Keeping your butt on the floor, reach forward with your torso and drape your body over your knees.

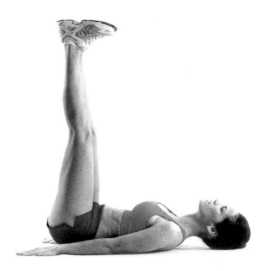

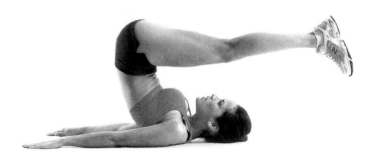

PLOW

Lie on your back, arms at your sides and legs straight up, so your body forms a 90-degree angle. Squeeze your abs, keep your legs straight, and bring your legs back overhead. Try to touch the floor with your toes. Keep your chin away from your chest.

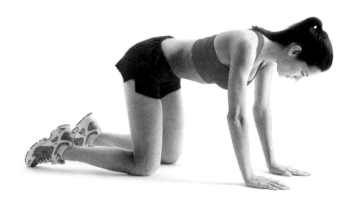

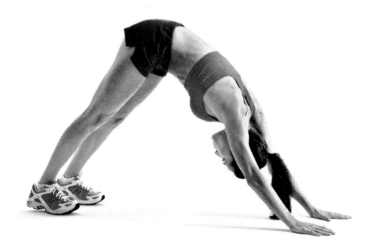

DOWNWARD DOG

Start on all fours with your hands shoulder-width apart and slowly lift your knees
off the floor. Shift your hips as far back as possible to lengthen your spine and
straighten your legs only to the extent that your spine can remain elongated.
The position looks like an inverted V.

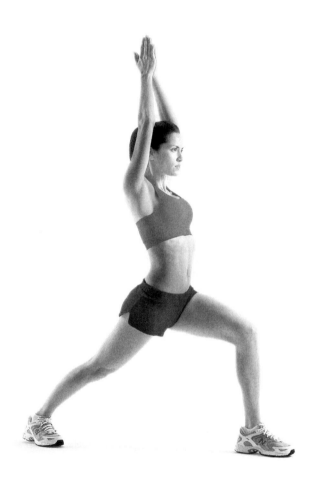

WARRIOR I

From downward dog, take one foot forward between your hands so that your forward thigh is parallel to the ground. Turn your back heel down and square your hips toward the front. Open up your chest by raising your arms over your head and putting your palms together. Lean your head back and lengthen your lower back by moving your tailbone toward the ground (keep your back leg straight). Hold, then switch sides.

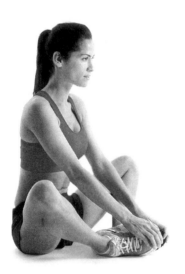
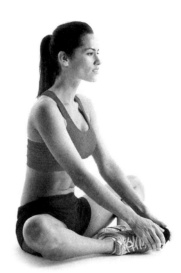

COBBLER'S POSE

Sit down on the floor or a yoga block or blanket with the soles of your feet pressed together. (You can keep your back pressed against a wall for additional support.) Drop your knees so your inside thighs open up comfortably.

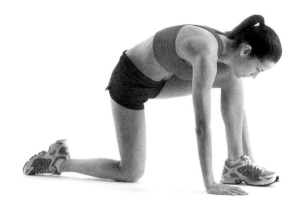

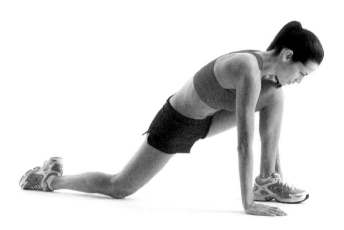

LUNGE

On all fours, step your left foot forward so your toes line up with your fingers and your knee is over your ankle. Next, slide your right leg behind you with your knee on the floor. Keep your spine long and straight and your shoulder blades down. To deepen the stretch, press your hips forward and down and your collarbones up. Breathe, switch sides, and repeat.

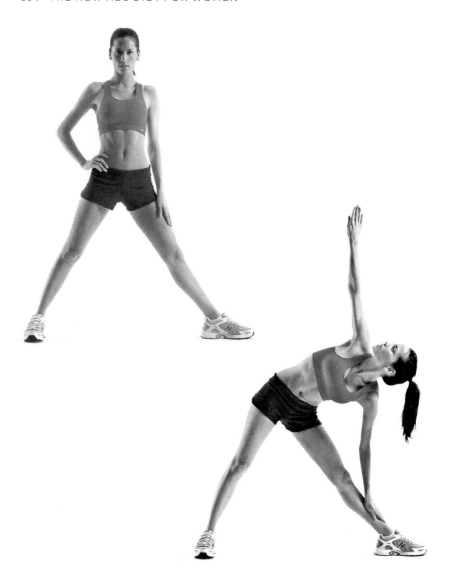

TRIANGLE POSE

Standing with your legs wider than shoulder-width apart, point your left toe to
the side and your right foot forward. Place your left hand on your left shin or ankle,
and your right hand on your right ribs. Then roll your torso open to the right so your
right shoulder lines up over your left shoulder. If you feel steady, lift your right arm
straight up toward the ceiling so it's in line with your left arm. Keep your spine
long and look up at your right arm. If this bothers your neck, gaze straight ahead.
Breathe, switch sides, and repeat.

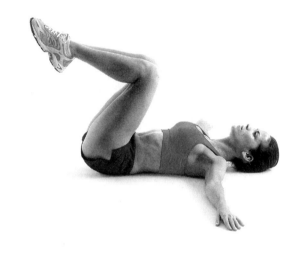

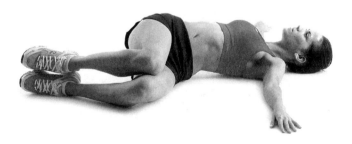

RECLINED TWIST

Lie on your back with your arms extended. Bring your knees to your chest at about a 45-degree angle. With an exhale, lower your knees to the left, keeping them stacked on top of each other. Hold, then switch sides.

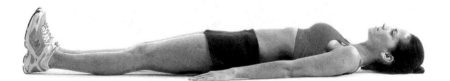

CLASSIC RELAXATION

Lie on the floor with your eyes closed. Let your arms rest to your sides, with your fingers relaxed. Let your legs relax. Take 10 seconds to breathe in and 10 seconds to breathe out. Continue as long as you like.

High-Intensity Posing

IF YOU'RE INTO mat work, then you know you can get a good calorie burn from stretching, bending, and twisting. An active sequence of yoga flows—a form called vinyasa—burns more than 450 calories an hour. These two flows provide a total-body burn. Repeat each one 5 to 10 times.

FLOW 1: CHAIR POSE
TARGETS: LOWER BODY

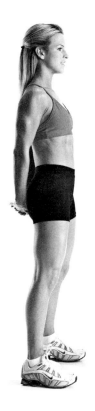
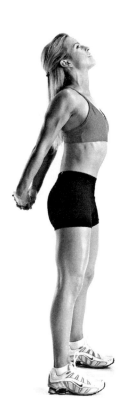

BACKBEND
Stand with your feet hip-width apart. Lace your fingers behind you (palms facing up). Inhaling, bend from your upper back, lift your chest, and press your shoulders down.

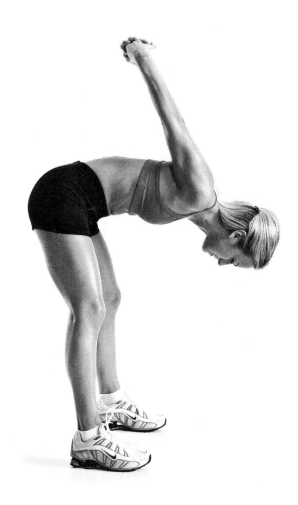

FORWARD BEND

Soften your knees and bend forward as you exhale, letting your torso hang in front of your thighs. Keeping your arms straight and fingers locked together, lift them up and over your head (ultimately reaching toward the floor in front of your feet).

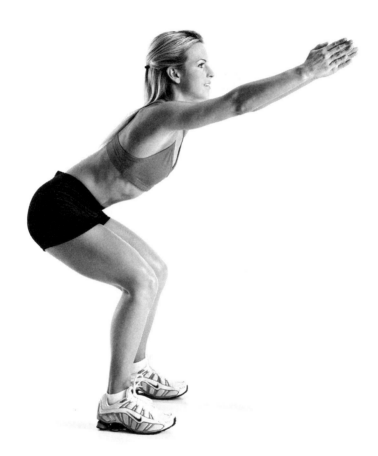

CHAIR

Inhale and bend your knees into a squat. Unlock and straighten your fingers, then separate your arms. When your thighs are nearly parallel to the floor, move your arms toward your ears. Keep your weight on your heels. Inhale, stand up, and lower your arms to your sides. Exhale.

FLOW 2: DOG POSE
TARGETS: UPPER BODY

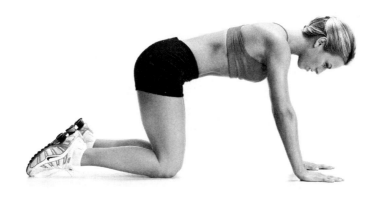

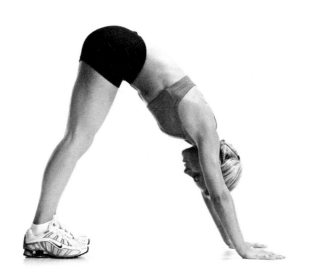

DOWNWARD DOG

Start on all fours with your hands shoulder-width apart and slowly lift your knees off the floor. Shift your hips as far back as possible to lengthen your spine, and straighten your legs only to the extent that your spine can remain elongated. The position looks like an inverted V.

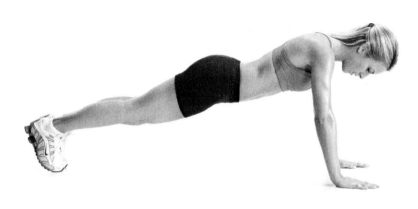

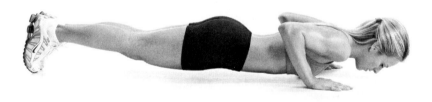

PLANK

Inhale as you shift forward into the top of a pushup position with your arms straight. Exhale, bend your elbows (keep them pointing back and hugging your body), and lower your body until your chest is on the ground.

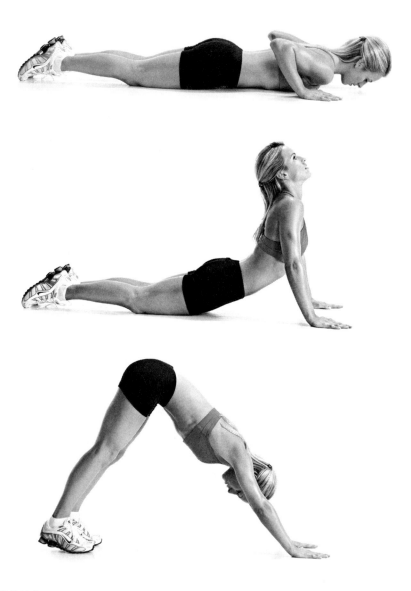

COBRA

Uncurl your toes so the tops of your feet are touching the ground, and press your tailbone down. Hug your elbows in as you inhale, straighten your arms (keep a slight bend), and lift your chest off the ground. Exhale as you gently release your body back to the ground. Inhale, curl your toes under, and press your hips up and back into downward dog. Exhale.

Buff-Body Yoga

IRON YOGA ISN'T a way to combine working out and doing chores. It's a workout that combines two popular forms of exercise into one total-body routine. Here's how it works: While you're lunging or balancing in a yoga pose, your legs and torso muscles are working hard to keep you upright. If you add a pair of dumbbells (2 to 5 pounds), suddenly your upper-body muscles are working, too, so that you get the benefits of a stronger lower body, greater flexibility, straighter posture, and reduced stress, along with stronger arms, shoulders, and back. Triathlete Anthony Carillo created Iron Yoga as a way to fit yoga into his grueling training schedule, but any level of exerciser can do the routine. If you're a yoga novice, practice the poses starting on page 344 without weights for 2 to 4 weeks until you feel comfortable, and then add dumbbells.

||||||||||||||||||||||||||||||||||||||||||||||||||||||||||||||||||||||||||||||||||||||||||||||||||||||||

Crunched for Time

Researchers at the University of Virginia found that it takes 250,000 crunches to burn a pound of fat. That's 100 crunches a day for 7 years. Chances are you can't wait that long. Still, in the quest for a flat stomach, you'll take an extra burn wherever you can get it, like these quick ways to burn 100 calories.

▶ Ride a stationary bike at 20 mph for 4 minutes 52 seconds.

▶ Shovel snow for 12 minutes.

▶ Walk uphill for 13 minutes.

▶ Rake leaves for 20 minutes.

▶ Give a full-body massage for 19½ minutes.

▶ Walk the dog for 23 minutes.

▶ Slow dance for 36 minutes.

▶ Tap your foot 9,351 times.

Iron Yoga Poses

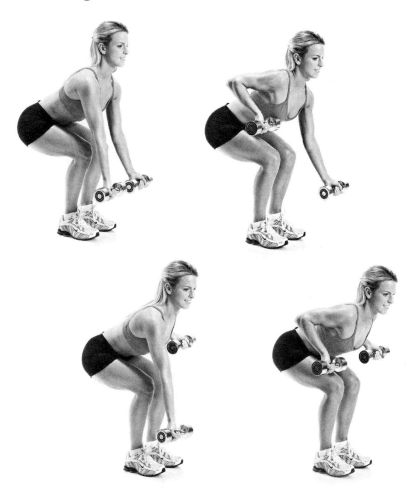

CHAIR POSE WITH ROW

With your feet together and a dumbbell in each hand, sit back until your thighs are almost parallel to floor. (Beginners don't have to go so low.) Keep your back flat and look at the floor about 2 feet in front of you. Rotate your palms up and press ends of dumbbells together; don't let arms touch knees. Without moving your left arm, inhale and bend your right elbow back toward the ceiling and pull the dumbbell toward your chest. Exhale and lower. Repeat with your left arm once. Repeat with both arms at the same time and hold for one static contraction. Lower and stand up.

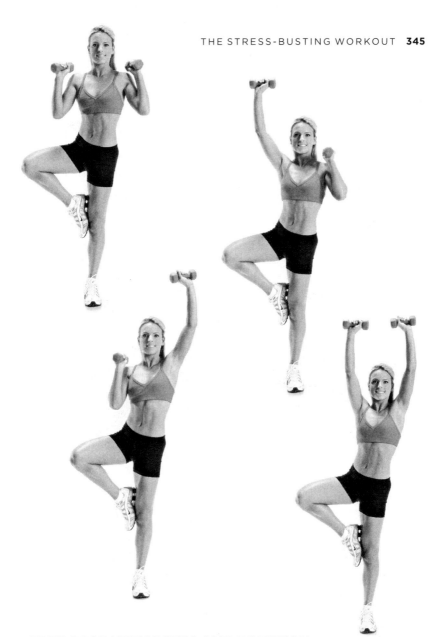

TREE POSE WITH PRESS AND ROTATION

Balancing on your left foot, place your right foot on the inside of your left thigh. (Beginners can place the foot on the inside of the calf or keep toes lightly touching floor.) Bring the dumbbells above your shoulders, palms facing in. Inhale and press the right dumbbell overhead, keeping your arm close to your ear. Then exhale and pull back down. Repeat with your left arm once, then with both arms at the same time, pressing the dumbbells together when overhead and holding for one static contraction. Lower and switch legs.

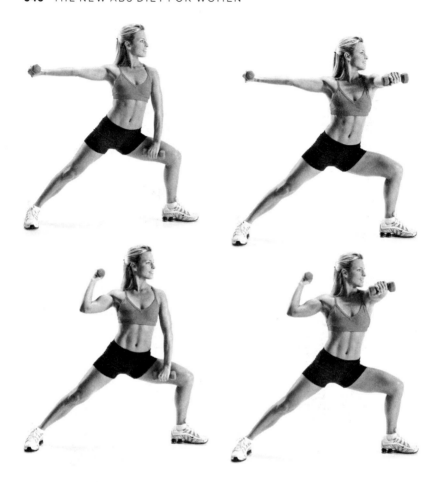

WARRIOR II WITH RAISE AND CURL

Step your right foot back about 4 feet. Turn your right foot out and rotate your torso to the right to square your hips and shoulders over the center of your body. Keep your left foot pointing and head looking straight ahead. Bend your left knee over your ankle until your thigh is about parallel to the floor. Raise your right arm behind you to shoulder height, palm up. Hold your left arm over your left knee, palm down. Inhale and raise the left dumbbell straight up in front to shoulder height. Exhale and lower the dumbbell. Do just once. Without moving your left arm, inhale and bend your right elbow, curling the dumbbell toward your shoulder (not shown). Exhale and press the dumbbell back to the starting position. Do just once. Raise your left arm and bend your right arm at the same time and hold for one static contraction. Return to the starting position and repeat with opposite legs and arms. Finish standing with feet together.

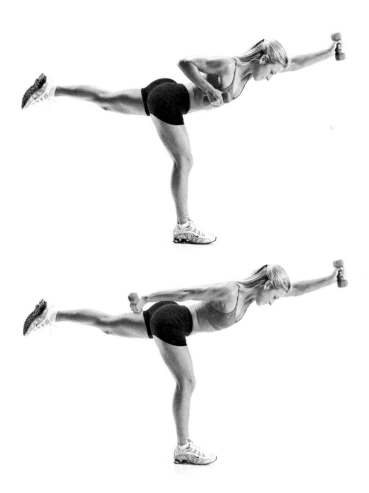

WARRIOR III WITH KICKBACK

Step your left foot back about 3 feet (not shown). Lean forward from your hips, bring the right dumbbell to your right armpit with elbow lifted, and raise the left dumbbell straight in front to shoulder height, palm facing in. Lift your left foot off the floor and extend your left leg straight back with toes pointed to form a straight line from left dumbbell to left toes. (Beginners can rest the extended arm on top of a chair for balance.) Inhale and extend your right arm, rotating the palm toward the ceiling, as you press the dumbbell behind you. Exhale and curl the dumbbell back toward your armpit. Do two reps, and then hold for one static contraction. Return to the starting position, lower your arms and leg, and repeat with your opposite leg raised, switching arms.

Pilates Moves

IT'S NO SECRET that staying in shape gets harder as you get older. (To prove it: In a University of Vermont study of women ages 20 to 60, researchers found that the oldest had 55 percent more belly fat than the youngest.) One of the ways to counter the effects of aging and too much potato salad is through the Abs Diet eating and exercise program. Abdominal exercises are one of the components that will help flatten and tone your stomach, but you don't have to be limited to the abdominal exercises I outlined earlier in the book. You can learn a lot from taking a Pilates class—a class that focuses on building and working all of the muscles in your core and torso.

One of the keys to Pilates training is to maintain what the experts call a neutral spine—that is, the position that keeps your abdominal muscles active but not too tight to allow an equal distribution of force throughout your torso. To find that position for yourself, locate a spot about 2 inches below your belly button. Now pull those muscles in and up—but not too hard. (It should feel like you're trying to squeeze into a pair of pants that's just a little too tight.) That's what a neutral spine feels like—and it's the position you should hold for all your moves. Pick four or five of these moves for the abdominal component of the Abs Workout, or just substitute one or two in your regular circuit.

Pilates Moves

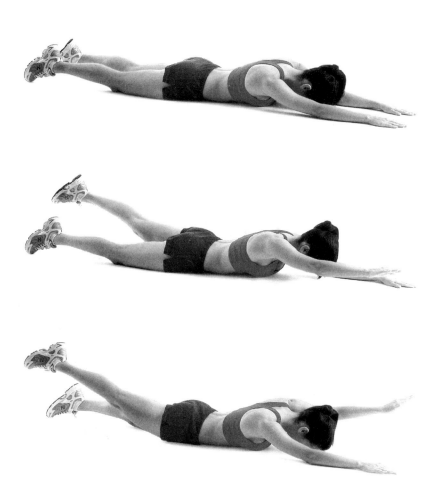

SWIMMING

Lie facedown on a mat or carpeted floor with your legs extended behind you.
Press your pelvis toward the floor and draw your navel toward your spine. Raise your
right arm and left leg as high as comfortably possible. Lift your head and chest off
the floor and begin to alternate your arms and legs in a rhythmic swimming motion,
inhaling and exhaling for 10 repetitions per side.

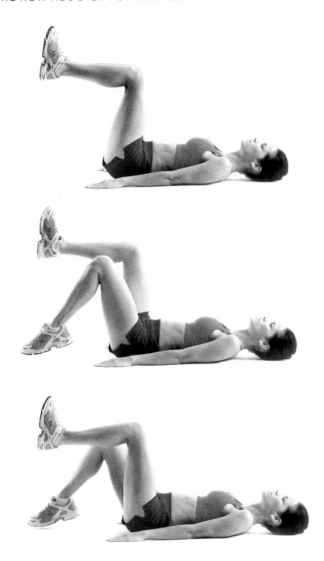

TOE DIP

Lie on your back with your legs bent at 90 degrees—thighs straight up and calves parallel to the floor. Rest your hands at your sides, palms down. Keep your abs contracted and press your lower back toward the floor. Inhale and lower your left leg for a count of two, moving only from your hip and dipping your toes toward the floor (without letting them touch it). Exhale and raise your leg back to the starting position for a count of two. Repeat with your right leg, and continue alternating until you've done 12 reps with each leg.

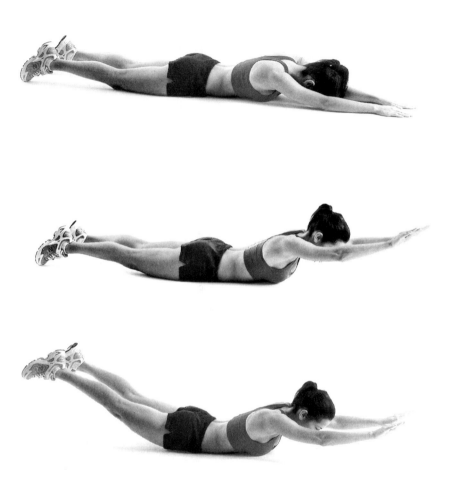

SWAN LIE

Lie facedown on a mat or carpeted floor with your legs extended behind you and the tops of your feet flat on the floor. With your arms extended in front of you, hands with palms down, raise your upper body, chest, and head. Then raise your legs. Pause, then lower your upper body, followed by your legs. Repeat 10 times.

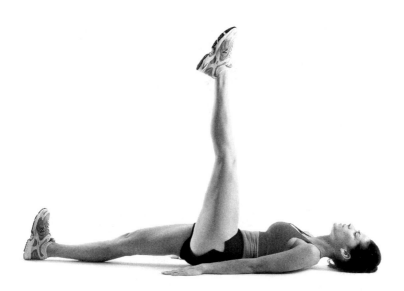

LEG CIRCLE

Lie on your back with your legs extended along the floor. Raise your left leg toward the ceiling, with toes pointed and hands at your sides, palms down. Hold for 10 to 60 seconds. Make a small circle on the ceiling with your left toes, rotating your leg from your hip. Inhale as you begin the circle and exhale as you finish. Keep your body as still as possible—no rocking—by tightening your abs. Do six circles, then reverse direction for six more. Repeat with the other leg.

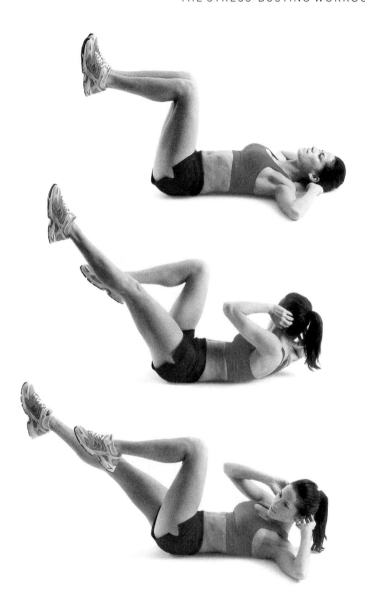

CRISSCROSS

Start as in the toe dip but with your hands behind your head, elbows out to the sides. Curl up to raise your head, neck, and shoulders off the floor. As you inhale, rotate your torso to the right, bringing your right knee and left shoulder toward each other and extending your left leg toward the ceiling in a diagonal line from your hips. As you exhale, rotate to the left, bringing your left knee toward your right shoulder and extending your right leg. That's 1 repetition; do 6.

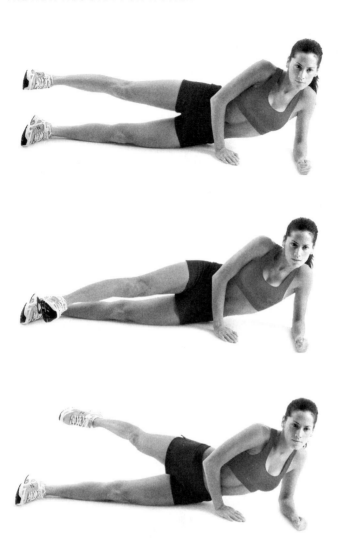

LEG KICK

Lie on your left side with your legs straight and together so your body forms one long line. Prop yourself up on your left elbow and forearm, lifting your ribs off the floor and your head toward the ceiling. Place your right hand lightly on the floor in front of you for balance. Raise your right leg to hip level and flex your foot so your toes are pointing forward. Exhale as you kick, swinging your right leg forward as far as comfortably possible and pulsing for two counts. Inhale, point your toes, and swing your leg back past your left leg. That's 1 rep. Do 6 without lowering your leg. Then switch sides and repeat.

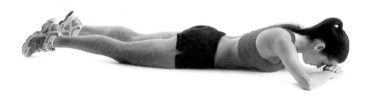

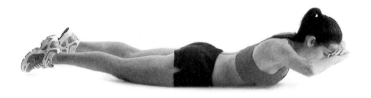

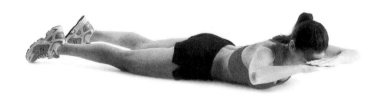

BACK EXTENSION WITH ROTATION

Lie on your stomach with your forehead on your hands, palms on the floor. Separate your feet to hip width. Pull your abs in. Raise your head, shoulders, and chest off the floor. Rotate your upper body to the right and back to center, then lower. Repeat to the left side, and continue alternating until you've done six rotations to each side.

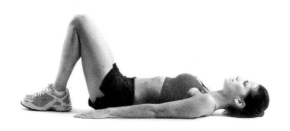

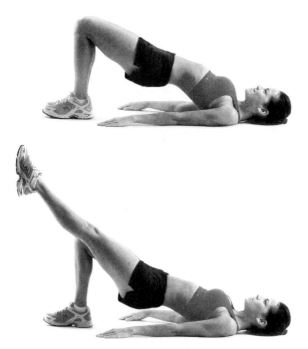

SHOULDER BRIDGE

Lie on your back with your knees bent, feet flat on the floor at a comfortable distance apart, heels close to your butt. Tighten your glutes and tilt your pelvis forward, raising your hips toward the ceiling slowly until your body forms a straight line from your shoulders to your knees. Keeping your hips aligned, lift your left foot off the floor and extend your leg straight out. Pause, then lower and repeat with the right leg. Then slowly lower your body back to the floor. Repeat 10 times.

|||||||||||||||||||||||||||||||||||||||||||||||||||||||||||||||||||||||||||||||||||||||||||||||||||||||||||

Get Energized

Sometimes, our bodies need the slow, calming pace of yoga or Pilates, but sometimes, when we're feeling especially sluggish, we need to be jump-started like a dead battery—with a jolt of energy that sends us rocketing through the day. For a 5-minute energy builder that will also burn a few calories, do high-intensity moves that get your blood flowing, your muscles stretched, and your mind ready to take on the children, the clients, or the clients who act like children.

Skip hops. Step forward with your left foot and as you land, hop into the air, bending your right knee in front. Land on your right foot and hop again. Do for 2 minutes.

March. March in place as quickly as possible, letting your arms swing naturally. Do for 30 seconds.

Jump rope. Do it for 30 seconds, landing softly on the balls of your feet. No rope? Mimic the motion without one.

One-leg hop. Stand on one foot, hands on hips. Jump straight up, landing softly with a bent knee. Do 15 seconds on each leg.

THE NEW ABS DIET MAINTENANCE PLAN

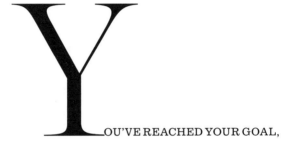OU'VE REACHED YOUR GOAL, and that's reason to celebrate. But it doesn't give you license to go back to breakfasts of leftover jalapeño poppers. However, you have earned a reprieve. You've built your body to churn fat and build lean muscle. With that base, you're at the point where your body is doing a lot of the work for you. Here's a primer for maintaining the body you've built.

SUBJECT	GUIDELINE
Diet basics	You've adjusted well, and you can continue eating six meals a day by focusing on the powerfoods—and the super ingredients, like protein, fiber, and whole-grain carbohydrates. Keep drinking smoothies regularly and adding a source of protein to every snack.
Cheating	You can up your cheating meal to a cheating day where you treat yourself to anything you want. Just keep it confined to 1 day rather than spreading it out over several meals on several days. That will increase the chances you'll stay focused and maintain good eating habits.

(continued)

SUBJECT	GUIDELINE
Exercise program	You're in maintenance mode now. Keep going with the program if you like, but you can also scale back to 1 or 2 days a week of strength training and 1 day a week of interval training. Research at the human performance laboratory at Ball State University has shown that lifters can maintain their muscle with just one workout a week.
Abdominal workout	Do a circuit of abdominal exercises before your strength training workouts. Move up to advanced exercises. Now that you can see your abs, you will want to increase the intensity. Still, for maximum growth, you shouldn't work your abs more than 2 or 3 days a week.

NUTRITIONAL VALUES OF COMMON FOODS

T HE TREND TOWARD LOW-carb diets has a lot of us eating plenty of fat and protein. But many of us are missing out on the valuable micronutrients found in whole grains, fruits, vegetables, and other foods that are verboten on a low-carb diet.

It might seem easier to ensure your daily value of nutrients by popping a multivitamin instead of eating a balanced diet. But there are two problems with nutrition that comes in a plastic container: First, multivitamins have no fiber, so this critical nutrient is missing if all you do is pop a pill for protection. Second, foods are loaded with plenty of nutrients beyond the standard vitamins C and E—and the importance of many of these nutrients, called phytochemicals, is only now being understood. "In a balanced diet, there are thousands of antioxidants. In pill form, you're just getting a few out of the thousands," says Edgar Miller, MD, PhD, of Johns Hopkins University in Baltimore.

To see how nutritionally complete your diet is, refer to the following chart for each food's vitamin and mineral values, and tally your total intake. If you come up short of the recommended dietary allowances (RDAs) for women, don't worry. Just eat more foods high in whatever vitamins or minerals you're lacking, and take a multivitamin/mineral supplement each day.

	VITAMIN A (MCG)	VITAMIN B₁ (THIAMIN) (MG)	VITAMIN B₆ (MG)	FOLATE (MCG)	VITAMIN C (MG)
RDAS FOR WOMEN	**700**	**1.1**	**1.3**	**400**	**75**
Almonds (1 ounce)	0	0.05	0.03	11	0
Apple (1 medium)	8	0.02	0.06	4	6
Apricot (1)	67	0.01	0.02	3	3.50
Artichoke (1 medium)	0	0.10	0.15	87	15
Asparagus (1 medium spear)	12	0.02	0.01	8	1
Avocado (1)	122	0.20	0.60	124	16
Bacon (3 slices)	0	0.08	0.07	0.40	0
Bagel (4")	0	0.15	0.05	20	0
Banana (1 medium)	7	0.04	0.40	24	10
Beans, baked (1 cup)	13	0.40	0.34	61	8
Beans, black (1 cup cooked)	1	0.40	0.12	256	0
Beans, kidney (1 cup cooked)	0	0.28	0.21	230	2
Beans, lima (½ cup cooked)	32	0.12	0.16	22	9
Beans, navy (1 cup cooked)	0.36	0.40	0.30	255	1.64
Beans, pinto (1 cup cooked)	0	0.17	0.16	294	1.37
Beans, refried (1 cup)	0	0.07	0.36	28	15
Beans, white (1 cup cooked)	0	0.20	0.17	145	0
Beef, ground lean (3 ounces)	0	0.06	0.24	7	0
Beer (12 ounces)	0	0.02	0.18	21	0
Beets (½ cup)	3	0.02	0.05	74	3
Blueberries (1 pint)	17	0.11	0.15	17	28
Bran, wheat (1 cup)	0	0.14	0.35	14	0
Bread, rye (1 slice)	0.26	0.14	0.02	35	0.13
Bread, white (1 slice)	0	0.11	0.02	28	0
Bread, whole grain (1 slice)	0	0.11	0.10	30	0.08

VITAMIN E (MG)	CALCIUM (MG)	MAGNESIUM (MG)	POTASSIUM (MG)	SELENIUM (MCG)	ZINC (MG)	CALORIES
15	1,000	320	4,700	55	8	
6	71	86	180	0	1	170
0.25	8	7	148	0	0.06	80
0.30	5	3.50	90	0.03	0.07	20
0.24	56	77	474	0.26	0.60	25
0.18	4	2	32	0.37	0.10	5
3	22	78	1,204	0.80	0.84	250
0.06	2	6	107	12	0.70	110
0.04	16	26	90	28	1	247
0.12	6	32	422	1	0.20	110
1.35	127	81	752	12	4	239
0.14	46	120	610	2	1.90	240
0.05	62	74	717	2	1.80	260
0.12	27	63	485	1.70	0.70	229
0.73	127	107	670	11	1.90	255
1.61	72	70	495	19	1.70	245
0	88	83	675	3	3	240
1.74	161	113	1,004	2.30	2.50	249
0.15	7	19	265	0	4	185
0	18	21	89	2.50	0.04	153
0.03	11	16	221	0.50	0.24	29
1.65	17	17	223	0.30	0.50	165
0.54	26	220	426	28	3	120
0.11	23	13	53	10	0.36	83
0.06	38	6	25	4.30	0.20	67
0.09	24	14	53	8	0.30	65

	VITAMIN A (MCG)	VITAMIN B₁ (THIAMIN) (MG)	VITAMIN B₆ (MG)	FOLATE (MCG)	VITAMIN C (MG)
RDAS FOR WOMEN	**700**	**1.1**	**1.3**	**400**	**75**
Breakfast sandwich, fast-food (bacon, egg, and cheese)	0	0.53	0.16	73	2
Brussels sprouts (½ cup)	60	0.08	0.14	47	48
Cake, coffee (1 piece)	20	0.10	0.03	27	0.11
Cake, frosted (1 piece)	10	0.01	0.02	7	0.04
Canadian bacon (2 slices)	0	0.40	0.20	2	0
Candy, nonchocolate (1 package)	0	0	0	0	0
Cantaloupe (1 medium wedge)	345	0.04	0.07	21	37
Carrot (1)	734	0.04	0.08	12	4
Cauliflower (1 cup)	2	0.06	0.22	57	46
Celery (1 cup, strips)	55	0.03	0.10	45	4
Cereal, whole grain, with raisins (½ cup)	3	0.16	0.10	22	0.55
Cheddar cheese (1 slice)	75	0.01	0.02	5	0
Chef's salad with no dressing (1½ cups)	146	0.40	0.40	101	16
Cherries, sweet, raw (1 cup)	30	0.07	0.05	5.80	10
Chicken, skinless (½ breast)	4	0.04	0.32	2	0.71
Chickpeas (1 cup cooked)	4	0.19	0.22	282	2
Chili with beans (1 cup)	87	0.12	0.30	59	4
Chips, potato, light (1 ounce)	0	0.05	0.22	8	3.40
Chocolate (1.45 ounces)	20	0.05	0.01	5	0
Cinnamon bun (1)	0	0.12	0	17	0.06
Citrus fruits and frozen concentrate juices (12 ounces)	7	0.17	0.30	31	324
Clams, fried (¾ cup)	101	0.11	0.07	41	11.25
Coffee (1 cup)	0	0	0	5	0
Collards (1 cup cooked)	1,542	0.08	0.24	177	35

VITAMIN E (MG)	CALCIUM (MG)	MAGNESIUM (MG)	POTASSIUM (MG)	SELENIUM (MCG)	ZINC (MG)	CALORIES
15	1,000	320	4,700	55	8	
0.60	160	25	211	36.0	2	441
0.34	28	16	247	1.17	0.26	28
0.11	76	10	63	9	0.25	180
0	18	14	84	1.40	0.30	239
0.16	5	10	181	11	0.80	137
0	0	0	0	0	0	230
0.05	9	12	272	0.40	0.18	24
0.40	20	7	195	0.06	0.15	35
0.08	22	15	303	0.60	0.30	25
0.33	50	14	322	0.50	0.16	17
0.40	33	70	207	10	1	195
0.08	204	8	28	4	0.90	114
0	235	49	401	37	3	267
0.20	21	16	325	0.90	0.09	90
0.08	6.50	16	150	11	0.50	130
0.60	80	79	477	6	2.50	269
1.46	120	115	934	3	5	220
0.62	10	18	285	2	0.17	142
0.83	78	26	153	2	0.83	230
0.48	10	3.60	19	5	0.10	418
0.24	85	68	1,336	1	0.41	186
0	71	16	366	33	1.60	560
0.05	2	5	114	0	0.02	2
1.67	266	38	220	1	0.50	61

	VITAMIN A (MCG)	VITAMIN B$_1$ (THIAMIN) (MG)	VITAMIN B$_6$ (MG)	FOLATE (MCG)	VITAMIN C (MG)
RDAS FOR WOMEN	700	1.1	1.3	400	75
Cookie, chocolate chip (1)	0.04	0.01	0.01	0.90	0
Corn (1 cup)	0.26	0.06	0.16	115	12
Cottage cheese, low-fat (1 cup)	25	0.05	0.15	27	0
Crackers (12)	0	0.17	0	0	0
Cranberry juice cocktail (1 cup)	1	0.02	0.05	0	90
Cream cheese (1 tablespoon)	53	0	0	2	0
Cucumber with peel (½ cup)	10	0.01	0.02	7	2.76
Doughnut (1)	17	0.10	0.03	24	0.09
Egg, whole (1 large)	84	0.03	0.06	22	0
Eggplant (1 cup)	4	0.08	0.09	14	1
English muffin, whole wheat (1)	0.09	0.25	0.05	36	0
Fig bar cookies (2 bars)	3	0.05	0.02	11	0.10
Fish, white (1 fillet)	60	0.26	0.50	26	0
French fries (10)	0	0.07	0.16	8	6
Fruit, dried (1 ounce)	208	0.01	0.05	1.1	1
Fruit juice, unsweetened (1 cup)	0	0.02	0.06	35	40
Garlic (1 clove)	0	0	0.04	0.09	0.90
Graham cracker (1 large rectangular piece)	0	0.03	0.01	6	0
Granola bar (1)	2	0.06	0.02	6	0.22
Grape juice (1 cup)	1	0.07	0.16	8	0.25
Ham (1 slice)	0	0.20	0.10	1	0
Hamburger, fast-food, with condiments and vegetables (1)	4	0.30	0.12	52	2
Hot dog, fast-food (1)	0	0.44	0.09	85	0.09
Ice cream (1 serving)	6	0.03	0.04	11	0.46
Jam or preserves (1 tablespoon)	0.20	0	0	2	2

VITAMIN E (MG)	CALCIUM (MG)	MAGNESIUM (MG)	POTASSIUM (MG)	SELENIUM (MCG)	ZINC (MG)	CALORIES
15	1,000	320	4,700	55	8	
0.26	2.50	3	14	0	0.06	63
0.15	8	44	343	1.54	1.36	120
0.02	138	11	194	20	0.86	180
0	28	12	48	2.40	0.20	155
0	8	5	46	0	0.18	137
0.04	12	1	17	0.40	0.10	51
0	7	6	75	0	0.10	8
0.90	21	9	60	4	0.30	230
0.50	25	5	63	15	0.50	74
0.40	6	11	122	0.10	0.12	35
0.26	101	21	106	17	0.61	134
0.21	20	9	66	1	0.12	111
0.39	51	65	625	25	2	168
0.12	4	11	211	0.20	0.20	100
0.31	11.82	11.13	226	0	0.14	69
0	160	9	154	0	0.20	117
0	5	0.75	12	0.40	0	4
0.05	3	4	19	1	0.10	59
0.32	15	24	82	4	0.50	117
0	23	25	334	0.25	0.13	154
0.10	2	5	94	6	0.50	30
0.42	126	23	251	20	2	512
0.10	108	27	190	29	2	242
0	72	19	164	1.65	0.40	133
0	4	0.80	15	0.40	0	56

	VITAMIN A (MCG)	VITAMIN B₁ (THIAMIN) (MG)	VITAMIN B₆ (MG)	FOLATE (MCG)	VITAMIN C (MG)
RDAS FOR WOMEN	**700**	**1.1**	**1.3**	**400**	**75**
Kale (1 cup)	955	0.07	0.11	18	33
Ketchup (1 tablespoon)	7	0	0.02	2	2
Kiwifruit (1 medium)	3	0.02	0.07	19	70
Lasagna, meat (7 ounces)	61	0.19	0.20	16	12
Lentils (1 cup cooked)	4.75	0.33	0.35	358	0.22
Lettuce, iceberg (1 cup)	8	0.02	0.03	31	2
Lettuce, romaine (½ cup)	81	0.02	0.02	38	7
Liver, beef (3 ounces)	8,042	0.16	0.86	215	1.62
Lunchmeat, salami (3 slices)	0	0.10	0.08	0.34	0
Macaroni and cheese (8 ounces)	48	0.25	0	0	0
Meat loaf (1 slice)	20	0.10	0.14	12	0.62
Melon, honeydew (1 cup)	5	0.07	0.16	34	32
Milk, fat-free (1 cup)	5	0.10	0.10	12	2
Milk, soy (1 cup)	0	0.15	0.16	40	0
Muffin, blueberry (1)	13	0.10	0.01	42	0.63
Mushrooms (1 cup sliced)	0	0.09	0.10	12	2
Nachos with cheese (6–8)	170	0.20	0.20	12	1
Nectarine (1)	23	0.05	0.03	7	7
Oatmeal (1 cup)	0.12	0.12	0.10	13	0
Olives (1 tablespoon)	1.70	0	0	0	0
Onion rings (10 medium)	0.98	0.10	0.07	64	0.68
Oyster (1 medium)	4.20	0.01	0.01	1.40	0.52
Pancakes (2)	7.60	0.16	0.07	28	0.15
Pasta with red sauce (4.5 ounces)	0	0.13	0.10	4	6
Peach (1 medium)	16	0.02	0.02	4	6
Peanut butter (2 tablespoons)	0	0.03	0.15	24	0
Peanuts (1 ounce)	0	0.12	0.07	41	0

VITAMIN E (MG)	CALCIUM (MG)	MAGNESIUM (MG)	POTASSIUM (MG)	SELENIUM (MCG)	ZINC (MG)	CALORIES
15	**1,000**	**320**	**4,700**	**55**	**8**	
1	180	23	417	1.17	0.23	39
0.20	3	3	57	0.04	0	15
1	26	13	237	0.15	0.10	50
0.94	220	41	372	28	3	318
2.97	37	71	731	5.54	2.51	230
0.02	11	4	84	0.28	0.10	8
0.04	9	4	69	0.10	0.06	5
0.43	5	18	300	31	4.50	162
0.05	1.34	2.86	63	4	0.54	150
0	102	0	111	0	0	415
0.10	43	22	295	0	4	231
0.04	11	18	403	1.24	0.16	61
0.10	301	27	406	5	1	83
0	80	60	440	3	0.90	100
0.47	32	9	70	6	0.30	158
0.10	5	10	355	8	0.70	15
0	311	63	196	18	2	296
1	8	12	273	0	0.23	70
0.26	19	51	175	0	1.43	150
0.14	7	0.30	0.67	0.08	0	10
0.39	86	19	152	3	0.41	370
0.12	6	7	22	9	13	41
0.65	96	15	133	10	0.30	173
1.40	41	13	207	11	0.66	216
0.70	6	9	186	0.10	0.17	70
0	12	51	214	2	1	190
2	15	50	186	2	1	165

	VITAMIN A (MCG)	VITAMIN B₁ (THIAMIN) (MG)	VITAMIN B₆ (MG)	FOLATE (MCG)	VITAMIN C (MG)
RDAS FOR WOMEN	**700**	**1.1**	**1.3**	**400**	**75**
Pear (1 medium)	1.60	0.02	0.05	12	7
Pepper, chile, raw (½ pepper)	21.6	0.03	0.23	10.35	65
Peppers, sweet (10 strips)	78	0.04	0.13	13	70
Pie, apple (1 piece)	37	0.03	0.04	32	4
Pizza, cheese (1 slice)	74	0.20	0.04	35	1
Pizza, vegetable (1 slice)	58	0.40	0.50	116	79
Plum (1)	21	0.03	0.05	1.45	6
Popcorn (1 cup)	0.80	0.02	0.02	2	0
Pork (3 ounces)	0	0.80	0.30	3	0
Potatoes, mashed (1 cup)	8.40	0.20	0.50	17	13
Potato salad (1 cup)	2.93	0.20	0.40	19	19
Potpie, chicken	256	0.30	0.20	41	2
Pretzels (10 twists)	0	0.30	0.07	103	0
Raisins (1.5 ounces)	0	0.05	0.08	1.28	2.30
Raspberries (10)	0.38	0.01	0.01	4	5
Rice, brown (1 cup)	0	0.20	0.30	8	0
Rice, white (1 cup)	0	0.03	0.15	5	0
Ricotta cheese, part skim (½ cup)	132	0.03	0.02	16	0
Salad dressing, light Italian (1 tablespoon)	0	0	0	0	0
Salmon (3 ounces)	9.84	0.20	0.71	22	0
Salsa (½ cup)	44	0.05	0.16	21	18
Sauerkraut (1 cup)	1.42	0.03	0.18	34	21
Sausage (1 link)	0	0.05	0.01	0.26	0
Shrimp (4 large)	0	0.01	0.03	0.77	0.48
Soft drink with caffeine (12 ounces)	0	0	0	0	0
Soup, cream of chicken (1 cup)	179	0.07	0.07	7	1.24

VITAMIN E (MG)	CALCIUM (MG)	MAGNESIUM (MG)	POTASSIUM (MG)	SELENIUM (MCG)	ZINC (MG)	CALORIES
15	**1,000**	**320**	**4,700**	**55**	**8**	
0.20	15	12	198	0.17	0.17	100
0.30	6	10	145	0.20	0.12	2
0.36	7	6.46	105	0	0	5
1.78	13	8	76	1	0.20	296
0	117	16	113	13	1	272
2	189	65	548	23	2	170
0	3	5	114	0.30	0.07	40
0	1	11	24	0.80	0.30	31
0.20	6	15	253	14	2	191
0.04	46	38	621	2	0.60	201
0.14	14	36	551	10	0.60	358
4	33	24	256	0.70	1	484
0.21	22	21	88	3	0.50	229
0.30	12	13	350	0.26	0.08	127
0.17	5	4	28	0.04	0.08	10
0.06	20	84	84	19	1	216
0.06	16	19	55	12	0.80	205
0.09	337	19	155	21	1.70	171
0	0	0	2	0.20	0	26
0.95	11	28	475	35	0.60	175
1.53	39	17	275	0.50	0.30	41
0.14	43	18	241	0.90	0.30	45
0.03	1.30	1.56	25	1.87	0.24	125
0	9	7	40	9	0.30	22
0	10	3	3	0.34	0	154
0.25	181	17	272	8	0.67	225

	VITAMIN A (MCG)	VITAMIN B₁ (THIAMIN) (MG)	VITAMIN B₆ (MG)	FOLATE (MCG)	VITAMIN C (MG)
RDAS FOR WOMEN	700	1.1	1.3	400	75
Soup, tomato (1 cup)	29.28	0.09	0.11	15	66
Soybeans (1 cup cooked)	14	0.47	0.10	200	31
Spaghetti with meatballs (1½ cups)	46	0.38	0.43	101	24
Spareribs (3 ounces)	1.91	0.26	0.22	3	0
Spinach (1 cup)	140	0.02	0.06	58	8
Steak (different cuts)	0	0.10	0.30	6	0
Strawberries (1 cup)	1.66	0.03	0.09	40	97
Submarine sandwich	71	1	0.10	87	12
Sunflower seeds (¼ cup)	5	0	0.28	82	0.50
Sweet potato (1)	350	0.09	0.25	9	19
Taco salad (1.5 cups)	71	0.10	0.20	83	4
Toaster pastry (1)	148	0.20	0.20	15	0
Tofu (4 ounces)	4.96	0.10	0.06	19	0
Tomato (1 medium)	26	0.02	0.05	9	8
Tuna salad (1 cup)	49	0.06	0.17	16	5
Turkey, skinless (½ breast)	0	0.16	2.26	31	0
Vegetable juice (1 cup)	188	0.10	0.30	51	67
Walnuts (1 cup)	37	0.27	0.70	82	4
Watermelon (1 wedge)	104	0.20	0.40	6	31
Wheat germ (½ cup)	0	0.20	0.40	81	0
Whey protein powder (2 teaspoons)	0	0	0	0	0
Wine, red (3.5 ounces)	0	0	0.03	2	0
Wine, white (3.5 ounces)	0	0	0.01	0	0
Yogurt, low-fat (8 ounces)	2	0.10	0.09	24	1.70

VITAMIN E (MG)	CALCIUM (MG)	MAGNESIUM (MG)	POTASSIUM (MG)	SELENIUM (MCG)	ZINC (MG)	CALORIES
15	1,000	320	4,700	55	8	
2	12	7	263	0.50	0.24	180
0.02	261	108	970	3	1.64	298
4	138	66	718	39	5	545
0.20	30	15	204	24	3	338
0.60	30	24	167	0.30	0.16	10
0.11	4	19	250	12	3.26	217
0.50	27	22	253	1	0.20	46
0	189	68	394	31	2.60	386
12	42	127	248	21.42	1.82	205
1.42	41	27	348	0.30	0.30	103
192	51	416	4	3	0	279
0.90	17	12	57	6.30	0.30	204
0.01	434	37	150	11	1	75
0.33	6	7	146	0	0.11	35
2	35	39	365	84	1	383
0.30	39	109	1,142	95	5	413
12	26	27	467	1	0.50	50
0	73	253	655	21	4.28	654
0.40	41	31	479	0.30	0.20	86
0	27	275	166	91	14	104
0	0	0	260	0	0	21
0	8	13	111	0.20	0.10	88
0	9	10	80	0.20	0.07	86
0	415	37	497	11	1.88	193

GLYCEMIC LOADS FOR SELECTED FOODS

Peanuts	1	All-Bran cereal	9
Low-fat yogurt, artificially sweetened	2	Grapefruit juice	9
		Hamburger bun	9
Carrots	3	Kidney beans, canned	9
Grapefruit	3	Lentil soup	9
Green peas	3	Oatmeal cookies	9
Fat-free milk	4	Sweet corn	9
Pear	4	American rye bread	10
Watermelon	4	Cheese tortellini	10
Beets	5	Frozen waffles	10
Orange	5	Honey	10
Peach	5	Lima beans, frozen	10
Plum	5	Low-fat yogurt, sweetened with sugar	10
Apple	6	Pinto beans	10
Kiwifruit	6	White bread	10
Tomato soup	6	Bran Chex cereal	11
Baked beans	7	Apple juice	12
Chickpeas, canned	7	Banana	12
Grapes	7	Kaiser roll	12
Pineapple	7	Orange juice	12
Whole-wheat bread	7	Saltine crackers	12
Popcorn	8	Bran flakes	13
Soy milk	8	Oatmeal	13
Taco shells	8		

Graham crackers	14	Total cereal	17
Special K cereal	14	Brown rice	18
Vanilla wafers	14	Fettuccine	18
Bran muffin	15	Angel food cake	19
Cheerios cereal	15	Cornflakes cereal	21
French bread	15	French fries	22
Grape-Nuts cereal	15	Jelly beans	22
Mashed potatoes	15	Macaroni	22
Shredded wheat cereal	15	Rice Krispies cereal	22
Bread stuffing mix	16	Couscous	23
Cheese pizza	16	Linguine	23
Whole-wheat spaghetti	16	Long-grain rice	23
Black bean soup	17	White rice	23
Blueberry muffin	17	Bagel	25
Corn chips	17	Baked potato	26
Doughnut	17	Spaghetti	27
Grape-Nuts Flakes cereal	17	Raisins	28
Instant oatmeal	17	Macaroni and cheese	32
Rice cakes	17	Instant rice	36
Sweet potato	17		

||||||||||||||||||||||||||||||||||||||||||||||||||||||||||||||||||||||||||||||||||||||||

How to Use This Chart

The numbers in this chart represent the glycemic loads (GLs) of common foods. The GL is the product of a food's glycemic index and the amount of carbohydrates available per serving. Essentially, the GL estimates the projected elevation in blood glucose caused by eating a particular food. The higher a food's GL, the higher it is likely to be in both calories and carbs, so try to center your meals around foods with a GL of 19 or less and shoot for a total GL of less than 120 for the whole day.

INDEX

Boldface page references indicate photographs.
Underscored references indicate tables or boxed text.